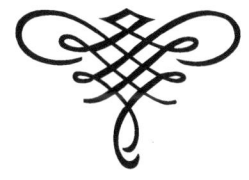

ULTIMATE GUIDE TO PLASTIC SURGERY

A Comprehensive Analysis of Procedures, Risks, Benefits, Costs, and Recovery Times for Men and Women

Dr. Samantha Reynolds

Copyright © 2023

Notice of Copyright

All rights reserved.

No part of this publication may be reproduced, stored in a retrieval system, stored in a database and / or published in any form or by any means, electronic, mechanical, photocopying, recording or otherwise, without the prior written permission of the publisher.

Authored by:
Dr. Samantha Reynolds

Printed in the United States of America

First Printing Edition, 2023
ISBN 9798863460161

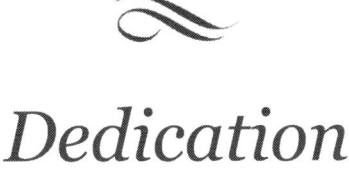

Dedication

To the lovers of beauty and aesthetics.

This book is dedicated to you.

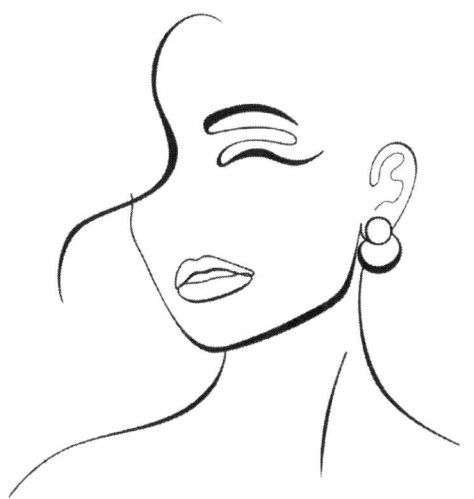

Table of Contents

INTRODUCTION 1

CHAPTER ONE 4

1. UNDERSTANDING PLASTIC SURGERY 4

What is Plastic Surgery? 4

The History of Plastic Surgery 6

Reasons for Considering Plastic Surgery 7

    Personal Satisfaction and Confidence 8

    Medical Necessity and Reconstruction 8

    Professional Pressures 8

    Body Image and Social Influence 8

    Aging Gracefully 9

    Health Benefits 9

Risks and Benefits of Plastic Surgery 9

    Benefits: More Than Skin Deep 10

    Risks: The Other Side of the Coin 11

Cost of Plastic Surgery 12

    Professional Fees 12

    Facility Costs 12

    Additional Costs 13

    Miscellaneous 13

Geographical Variations 13

Payment Plans and Financing 13

Insurance Caveats 14

Types of Plastic Surgery Procedures 14

Facial Procedures 14

Body Procedures 15

Gender-Specific Procedures 15

Reconstructive Procedures 16

Minimally Invasive Options 16

Cutting-Edge Procedures 17

Common Myths About Plastic Surgery 18

#1 Plastic Surgery is Purely Cosmetic 18

#2 It's Only for the Wealthy 18

#3 Results Last Forever 18

#4 Recovery is a Walk in the Park 19

#5 It's a 'Vain' Choice 19

#6 Any Doctor Can Do It 19

#7 It's a Quick Fix for Body Issues 19

#8 It's Only for Women 20

#9 It's Only for Older People 20

CHAPTER TWO 22

2. COSMETIC PLASTIC SURGERY FOR WOMEN 22

Breast Augmentation 22

What is Breast Augmentation? 23

Implants or Fat Transfer: What's Your Style? 23

Setting Expectations: What Can It Do For You? 23

Pre-Surgical Preparations: Get Set Go 24

A Closer Look At The Operation 24

Post-Operation: The Recovery Timeline 24

Longevity: How Long Do Results Last? 24

Breast Lift 25

A breast lift is what? 25

How Does It Differ From Augmentation? 25

To Lift or Not to Lift: Are You a Candidate? 25

The Method Behind the Magic: Surgical Techniques 26

Recovery and Aftercare 26

Liposuction 26

The Science and the Art: Techniques Involved 27

Me, Myself, and Lipo: Who Needs It? 27

Price Tag and Piggy Banks: What Will It Cost? 27

Post-Surgery and Peace 28

Tummy Tuck 28

Choosing Your Path: Types of Tummy Tucks 28

Am I the One? Identifying Candidates 29

Investing in You: Let's Talk Money 29

The Aftermath: Recovery and What to Expect 29

The Unveiling: Long-term Results and Upkeep 30

Brazilian Butt Lift (BBL) 30

The Core Principle: Fat Transfer 30

To BBL or Not to BBL: Ideal Candidates 30

What Will It Cost? 31

Charting the Road to Recovery 31

Playing the Long Game: Sustaining the Results 31

Facelift 32
A Facelift in a Nutshell 32
Differences From Non-Surgical Treatments 32
Who Makes the Cut? Ideal Clients 32
Price Tag: What's the Damage? 33
Navigating the Aftermath: Recovery 33
Maintaining Your Youth: Longevity of Results 33

Rhinoplasty 34
What is a rhinoplasty exactly? 34
Distinguishing Cosmetic and Functional Rhinoplasty 34
Who's In? Ideal Candidates for Rhinoplasty 34
How Deep is the Dent in Your Wallet? 35
The Path to Your New Nose: Surgical Procedures 35
Healing and Aftercare: The Long Road to Recovery 35

Eyelid Surgery 36
What is Eyelid Surgery? 36
Upper Eyelid vs Lower Eyelid Surgery 36
Who Should Consider Eyelid Surgery? 36
Is Your Wallet Ready? 37
Procedure Specifics: What to Expect 37
After the Cuts: Recovery Insights 37

Lip Augmentation 38
What is Lip Augmentation? 38
Types of Lip Fillers 38
Are You a Good Fit for Lip Augmentation? 38
What's the Price Point? 39
The Procedure: An Overview 39
Recovery and Longevity: What Comes After 39

The End Game: Managing Expectations 39

Cheek Augmentation 40

What Exactly is Cheek Augmentation? 40

Surgical vs. Non-Surgical: Choices Abound 40

Are You a Candidate for Cheek Augmentation? 40

What's the Damage? 41

The Procedure Unveiled 41

Post-Procedure 41

Maintaining the Look 41

Results: Keep it Realistic 42

Botox and Fillers 42

The wrinkle whisperer, Botox 42

Fillers: The Volume Vendors 42

Pick Your Potion: Botox or Fillers? 43

Cost Comparison: What's the Dent in the Wallet? 43

Procedure Particulars 43

Recovery and Risks: Short and Sweet 43

Longevity of Results: Temporary but Repeatable 44

The Right Provider: Your Aesthetic Ally 44

Laser Treatments 44

The ABCs of Lasers 45

Different Lasers, Different Gains 45

Cost and Commitment 45

The Procedure and What to Expect 45

Short-Term and Long-Term Effects 46

Safety and Potential Side Effects 46

Aftercare is a Must 46

CHAPTER THREE 48

3. RECONSTRUCTIVE PLASTIC SURGERY FOR WOMEN 48

Breast Reconstruction **49**
    The Rundown on Breast Reconstruction 49
    Timing is Everything: Immediate vs. Delayed 49
    The Surgical Playbook: Techniques Explored............................49
    Insurance and Costs: The Financial Side 50
    The Recovery Roadmap 50
    Longevity and Maintenance: What Comes Next? 50
    Soul Food: Emotional and Psychological Impact.....................50

Cleft Lip and Palate Repair **51**
    The Fundamentals: What is Cleft Lip and Palate Repair? 51
    Types of Clefts and their Classification 51
    Treatment Stages: A Phased Approach 52
    Surgical Techniques and Innovations..52
    Impact on Feeding and Speech 52
    Financial and Insurance Considerations 52
    Emotional and Psychological Bearings 53
    Long-Term Outlook and Care...53

Scar Revision..**53**
    What is Scar Revision? 54
    Types of Scars and Their Complexity 54
    Surgical Procedures: A Toolbox of Techniques........................54
    Risks and Considerations...54
    Post-Surgery: The Recovery Timeline 55
    Insurance and Cost Factors...55
    Emotional and Psychological Impacts..55
    The Long-term Prognosis 55

Burn Reconstruction **56**

What is Burn Reconstruction? 56

Classification of Burns 56

The Stages of Reconstruction 56

Skin Grafts and Beyond 57

Risks and Challenges 57

Finances and Insurance 57

The Emotional Angle 57

Long-term Outlook 58

Vaginal Rejuvenation 58

What Exactly is Vaginal Rejuvenation? 58

Who Can Benefit? 59

Understanding the Procedures 59

The Crucial Role of Consultation 59

Risks and Side Effects 60

A Word on Finances 60

Emotional and Psychological Impact 60

Aftercare and Longevity 60

Tissue Expander Procedures 61

The 'What' of Tissue Expanders 61

How Does It Work? 61

Who's a Candidate? 62

Procedure Techniques 62

Risks and Complications 62

What to Expect Post-Procedure 62

Cost Factors 63

C H A P T E R   F O U R 65

4. COSMETIC PLASTIC SURGERY FOR MEN 65

Hair Transplant 65
Understanding Hair Transplants 66
Is It Right For You? 66
Techniques and Procedures 66
Financial Implications 66
Risks and Side Effects 67
Long-Term Results 67
Emotional Uplift 67
Post-Op Care 67

Abdominal Etching 68
The Basics of Abdominal Etching 68
Who's the Ideal Candidate? 68
The How-to: Surgical Procedure 69
Financial Commitment 69
Potential Risks 69
After the Cut: Recovery and Results 69
Lifestyle Impact 70

Jawline Enhancement 70
The Essence of Jawline Enhancement 70
Candidate Credentials 71
Procedural Steps 71
Fiscal Aspects 71
Consider the Risks 71
Journey of Recovery 72
Impact on Self-Image 72

Pectoral Implants 72
What are Pectoral Implants? 73
Who Stands to Benefit? 73

The Process 73
Budgetary Matters 73
Risk Factors 74
What to Expect After Surgery 74
Long-term Results and Self-Image 74

Liposuction 75
What is Liposuction? 75
Who's an Ideal Candidate? 75
How It's Done 75
Price Tag and Financing 76
Risks and Recovery 76
Long-lasting Impact 76
Mind the Mirror 76

Penis Enhancement 77
What Is Penis Enhancement? 77
The Right Candidate: Who Stands to Benefit? 77
Techniques Explored 78
Financial Aspects 78
Risks and Aftercare 78
Longevity of Results 78
Societal and Psychological Impacts 79

Gynecomastia Surgery 79
Defining Gynecomastia Surgery 79
Why Opt for Surgery? 80
Are You a Candidate? 80
Types of Procedures 80
What to Expect Post-Surgery 80
Cost Considerations 81

 Risks and Complications 81
 Lasting Impact 81

Botox and Fillers **81**
 Understanding Botox and Fillers 82
 Why the Growing Interest Among Men? 82
 Who's a Candidate? 82
 Different Products, Different Goals 83
 What About Risks? 83
 After the Procedure 83
 Let's Talk Budget 83

Laser Treatments **84**
 The What and How of Laser Treatments 84
 Why Men Are Opting for Lasers 84
 Suitability: Is It for You? 85
 Safety Concerns and Risks 85
 The Price Tag: What to Expect 85
 Post-Procedure Life 86

CHAPTER FIVE 88

5. RECONSTRUCTIVE PLASTIC SURGERY FOR MEN 88

Male Breast Reduction **88**
 What Male Breast Reduction Is All About 89
 What Triggers the Need? 89
 Getting Through the Pre-Surgery Maze 89
 Operational Tactics: The Procedure 90
 Recovery: The Road to Your New Self 90
 Cost and Insurance Coverage 90
 Long-Term Outcomes: Embrace the Change 91

Scar Revision 91
The Anatomy of Scar Revision 91
Why Consider Scar Revision? 92
Preparing for the Procedure 92
The Nuts and Bolts: Procedure Insights 92
Journey to Recovery 93
Financial Considerations 93
Sustaining the Results 93

Burn Reconstruction 94
The Anatomy of Burn Reconstruction 94
Why Burn Reconstruction? 94
Pre-Operative Evaluation 94
Behind the Scalpel: The Procedures 95
The Recovery Voyage 95
A Financial Palette 95
Longevity of Results 96

Earlobe Repair 96
The Why of Earlobe Repair 96
The Anatomy of the Repair 97
Procedure Nuances 97
Road to Recovery 97
Financial Footnote 97
The Legacy of Earlobe Repair 98

Hand Surgery 98
Why Opt for Hand Surgery? 98
The Types and Techniques 99
Navigating the Surgical Maze 99
Post-Op Pathway 99

The Economics of Hand Surgery 100
The Lingering Impact 100

Cleft Lip Repair in Men **100**
The Groundwork: What Is Cleft Lip in Men? 101
Why Choose Repair? 101
The Procedural Landscape 101
Life After the Knife: Recovery and Beyond 102
Cost Considerations 102
The Long Game: Reaping the Rewards 102

CHAPTER SIX 104

6. AESTHETIC DERMATOLOGY TREATMENTS 104

Mole Removal **105**
The Nature of Moles: Harmless or Cause for Concern? 105
Why Mole Removal? 105
Your Options Unveiled: Types of Mole Removal Techniques 106
Anticipating the Journey: Pre-Procedure Consultation 106
The Recovery Narrative 106
Pocket Impact: What Does Mole Removal Cost? 106

Age Spot Removal **107**
Age Spots 107
Deciding on Age Spot Removal 108
Techniques for Age Spot Removal 108
The Prep Work 108
Post-Treatment Care and Recovery 108
Cost Factor 109

Chemical Peels **109**

- Unveiling the Core of Chemical Peels 109
- A Solution for Every Skin Type 110
- Your Candidacy for the Procedure 110
- The Skin's Intermission: Prepping and Post-care 110
- Let's Talk Dollars: The Cost Aspect 111
- The Ticking Clock: Longevity of Results 111

PRP Therapy 111
- Unpacking the PRP Acronym 112
- The How-To of PRP Therapy 112
- Tailoring the Treatment 112
- Who Should Consider PRP? 112
- The Post-Procedure Phase 113
- Investment Breakdown 113
- Results' Lifespan 113

Laser Hair Removal 114
- Understanding the Laser Lingo 114
- From Consultation to Calibration 114
- The In-Office Experience 115
- Spotlight on Suitability 115
- Post-Procedure Protocol 115
- Zooming in on Costs 115
- The Long View 116

Cellulite Treatment 116
- What is Cellulite? 116
- Types of Treatments 117
- Non-Surgical Routes: How They Work 117
- Invasive Treatments: Going Under the Knife 117
- Who's the Best Candidate? 117

The Price of Perfection: What Will It Cost? 118

A Realistic Perspective: What to Expect 118

RF Microneedling **118**

Understanding the Procedure 119

Setting it Apart from Standard Microneedling 119

Who Should Consider It? 119

What's the Downtime? 120

The Financial Angle 120

CHAPTER SEVEN 122

7. PLASTIC SURGERY FAQS 122

What is the Difference Between Cosmetic and Reconstructive Plastic Surgery? **123**

Cosmetic Surgery: The Aesthetic Approach 123

Reconstructive Surgery: The Functional Fix 123

The Diverging Roads 123

What Are the Most Common Plastic Surgery Procedures? **124**

Breast Augmentation 124

Liposuction 124

Rhinoplasty 124

Tummy Tuck 124

Eyelid Surgery 125

Botox and Fillers 125

Hair Transplant 125

Brazilian Butt Lift (BBL) 125

Facelift 125

Am I a Good Candidate for Plastic Surgery? **126**

    Physical Health 126

    Psychological Wellness 126

    Skin Quality 126

    Lifestyle Choices 127

    Financial Readiness 127

    Individual Goals 127

    Long-term Commitment 127

What Should I Look for in a Plastic Surgeon? 128

    Board Certification 128

    Specialization 128

    Reviews and Reputation 129

    Before and After Photos 129

    Consultation Experience 129

    Hospital Privileges 129

    Cost 130

    Postoperative Care 130

What Are the Risks Associated With Plastic Surgery? 130

    Anesthesia Complications 131

    Infections 131

    Bleeding and Hematoma 131

    Scarring 131

    Nerve Damage 132

    Surgical Errors 132

    Emotional Toll 132

    Long-Term Complications 132

    Financial Strain 132

What is the Recovery Period of Different Plastic Surgery Procedures? 133

Breast Augmentation 133

Tummy Tuck: The Long Haul 133

Brazilian Butt Lift (BBL): Sit with Caution 134

Liposuction: It Varies 134

Rhinoplasty: A Nose by Any Other Name 134

Hair Transplant: Not a Quick Fix 134

Eyelid Surgery: Keep Those Eyes Closed 134

Chemical Peels: Surface vs Deep 135

Abdominal Etching: Quicker than You'd Think 135

PRP Therapy: Almost Instant 135

How Long Do the Results Last for Each Procedure? 135

Breast Augmentation: A Decade or More 136

Tummy Tuck: A Lifelong Commitment 136

Brazilian Butt Lift (BBL): Long-lasting but Not Forever 136

Liposuction: Permanent Fat Removal, Conditional Results 136

Rhinoplasty: Nearly Permanent 136

Hair Transplant: Differing Durabilities 137

Eyelid Surgery: A Decade of Youthful Eyes 137

Chemical Peels: From Months to Years 137

Abdominal Etching: Years with Caveats 137

PRP Therapy: Highly Variable 137

Facelift: Up to a Decade 138

Botox and Fillers: Temporary Satisfaction 138

What Plastic Surgery Procedures Leave Permanent Scars? 138

Unavoidable But Hidden: Tummy Tuck 138

Breast Augmentation and Lift: Scars With Options 139

Rhinoplasty: Minimal but Present 139

Facelift: Craftily Concealed 139

Hair Transplant: Tiny Dots or a Line 139

Liposuction: Small But Permanent 139

Brazilian Butt Lift: Nearly Invisible 140

Cleft Lip and Palate Repair: Unavoidable but Improved 140

Scar Revision: Irony of Sorts 140

Burn Reconstruction: Scars Changing Scars 140

How Much Does Plastic Surgery Cost Depending on the Procedure? 141

Tummy Tuck 141

Breast Augmentation 141

Rhinoplasty 141

Facelift 142

Hair Transplant 142

Liposuction 142

Brazilian Butt Lift 142

Cleft Lip and Palate Repair 142

Scar Revision 142

Burn Reconstruction 143

Botox and Fillers 143

Can I Undergo Plastic Surgery if I Have a Pre-existing Medical Condition? 143

Medical Evaluation 143

Chronic Conditions 144

Weight Concerns 144

Medication Adjustments 144

Mental Health 144

Minor Conditions 145

Financial Considerations 145

Final Clearance 145

CONCLUSION 147

REFERENCES 152

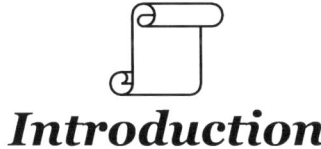

Introduction

You're thinking of getting cosmetic surgery, or perhaps you're just interested. Whatever the case may be, you're at the right place. Plastic surgery is actually a field that predates civilization itself and is sometimes thought of as the exclusive province of Hollywood stars and influential people. We're not kidding when we say that primitive versions of plastic surgery were practiced by ancient Egyptians. Don't worry though; the field has advanced greatly since then.

Plastic surgery nowadays is about more than simply appearance; it's also about confidence, reconstruction, and, for some people, a new beginning. Whether you're considering a stomach tuck, reconstructive surgery after an accident, or simply thinking about the complicated world of Botox and fillers, this book will take you on an enlightening trip covering everything you need to know.

We're not here to dissuade you from getting surgery or to convince you to do it. We want to give you thorough, unbiased information so you can make an informed choice. Think of this manual as a reliable buddy who has already completed all the research for you.

What can you anticipate from this guide, then? We'll begin by explaining the various categories of plastic surgery, both elective and necessary. We'll also help you make sense of the differences between the surgical alternatives for men and women. Have inquiries that you're afraid to ask anyone, let alone Google? We'll answer all of your questions as well as we progress through each chapter. Finally, we'll discuss under-discussed but crucial issues including mental health issues and post-surgery recuperation.

If you're unfamiliar with this subject, don't worry; we've avoided medical language whenever possible in order to make this information simple to understand. The content is enlightening for medical experts and includes data and study citations to support the information.

So let's start on this enlightening adventure right away. By the time you finish reading this book, you'll have the information you need to choose wisely while having plastic surgery, or you'll only know enough to impress everyone around you.

CHAPTER ONE

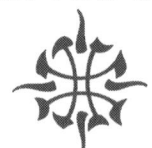

1. *Understanding Plastic Surgery*

Understanding the basics of this medical field is crucial before we start the process of changing our bodies through plastic surgery. To make wise selections, we must educate ourselves on all aspects of plastic surgery, from its origins and development to the different kinds of operations that are offered. This chapter will go into plastic surgery, discussing the motivations behind these procedures, the dangers and advantages, and the financial implications. We may better explore the options accessible to us and make decisions that are in line with our individual objectives and desires by developing a deeper awareness of plastic surgery.

What is Plastic Surgery?

When people hear the word "plastic surgery," they frequently picture celebrities with flawlessly youthful faces or Instagram influencers. The core of plastic surgery, however, goes well beyond the gloss and glamour, delving into the fields of medicine, art, and psychological well-being.

Let's begin with a straightforward definition. A specialist area of medicine known as "plastic surgery" focuses on changing, reconstructing, or repairing the human body. The word plastic has nothing to do with the Greek word plastikos, which means "to mold" or "to shape." In actuality, the field has a long and illustrious history, developing through the years from primitive suturing methods to the complex techniques we see today.

As diverse as the treatments themselves, the reasons people choose to get plastic surgery can also vary. Some people use it to improve their appearance; consider nose jobs, breast augmentations, and, yes, those Botox injections that reduce wrinkles. But plastic surgery also includes reconstructive treatments, so it's not only about improving your appearance. These operations are used to correct facial and physical deformities brought on by sickness, burns, congenital defects, or trauma. Reconstructive surgery tries to restore a damaged structure's functionality and give it a more 'normal' appearance.

Plastic surgery, whether aesthetic or reconstructive, has an essential component that is frequently disregarded: it does not provide a universally effective treatment. In order to practice in this discipline, medical personnel need to have a thorough awareness of each patient's individual physiology in addition to an artistic sense of balance and proportion. The path to the operating room is not merely transactional; it frequently entails numerous consultations, psychological assessments, and a thorough discussion of the advantages and disadvantages.

The History of Plastic Surgery

Contrary to popular belief, plastic surgery is not a recent phenomena. Its ancient origins are distinguished by innovations and developments that depict an engrossing tale of human ingenuity.

Around 600 BCE in ancient India, the first examples of treatments resembling plastic surgery were first documented. The surgical procedures for replacing noses and ears that had been lost as a result of punishment or battle were methodically described in the medical classic "Sushruta Samhita" (*Singh, 2017*). Ancient surgeons showed a startling level of skill in completing these reconstructive surgery using skin transplants from various regions of the body.

Imagine yourself in ancient Rome, when doctors would repair the face wounds suffered by gladiators, using crude but efficient methods to mend broken jaws and noses. The Romans experimented with cosmetic improvements as well, though not with the wide range of possibilities we're used to today (*Development Of Plastic Surgery - Pubmed, 2015*) .

Plastic surgery suffered a great deal of setbacks during the Middle Ages (*Development of Plastic Surgery - Pubmed, 2015*). Any medical procedures were forbidden due to superstitions and religious prohibitions. Nevertheless, anatomical research and surgical techniques gained popularity again throughout the Renaissance. Plastic surgery saw a resurgence of interest thanks to this period's scientific enthusiasm.

The horrific battles paradoxically contributed to the development of the field in the late 19th and early 20th centuries. The terrible damage that surgeons encountered required creative remedies. Reconstructive surgery became crucial in the treatment of injured troops as the idea of skin grafting was developed. Modern surgical methods were developed as a result of these experiences.

Plastic surgery has developed recently into a multidisciplinary field that makes use of cutting-edge technology. The field today functions at the crossroads of science, art, and technology, from laser-assisted operations to 3D-printed facial prosthesis. Additionally, it has divided into sub-specialties including reconstructive surgery, which focuses on functional restoration, and aesthetic surgery, which emphasizes cosmetic modifications.

Additionally, the conversation about plastic surgery is evolving. It's no longer stigmatized or cloaked in secrecy like it formerly was. In today's society, when both sexes freely share their experiences, plastic surgery is increasingly seen as a means of enhancing personal freedom.

Reasons for Considering Plastic Surgery

It's not unusual to want to alter one's look or fix a perceived imperfection; it's woven into the fabric of human existence. However, the reasons people choose to have plastic surgery are just as diverse as the people who visit the doctor. These motives frequently walk a fine line between medical need and aesthetic desires, each with its own set of complications and results.

Personal Satisfaction and Confidence

Many people seek plastic surgery because they want to feel more satisfied about themselves and have more confidence. These people seek positive transformation and a revitalized feeling of self, whether it be a belly tuck to get back to their pre-pregnancy bodies or a rhinoplasty to improve face symmetry.

Medical Necessity and Reconstruction

People who have experienced trauma can frequently find a lifeline through reconstructive surgery. Plastic surgery is frequently chosen as a means of functional restoration by accident victims, cancer patients, or people with congenital problems. The distinction between "want" and "need" becomes hazy in certain situations, emphasizing the significant influence plastic surgery has on quality of life.

Professional Pressures

A growing number of decisions now involve professional demands thanks to the development of social media and the visual culture it promotes. Actors, influencers, and even experts in fields like real estate and marketing who work in the public eye can think about plastic surgery to keep up their competitive edge.

Body Image and Social Influence

Cultural beauty standards have a significant impact on how people perceive themselves, frequently enhanced by social media. Although the effect isn't always bad, it does lead some people to seek out plastic surgery as a way to conform to social norms.

Aging Gracefully

Plastic surgery can be a tempting alternative for the elderly demographic to delay the unavoidable effects of aging. In order to regain a more youthful appearance and so boost their confidence, procedures including facelifts, brow lifts, and eyelid surgeries are frequently requested.

Health Benefits

The advantages to your health that come with particular operations are less talked about but no less significant. Chronic back pain can be relieved with a breast reduction, and mobility and skin infections can be prevented by eliminating extra skin following large weight loss (*MBBS, 2018*).

We can obtain a more detailed picture of why plastic surgery appeals to such a wide spectrum of people by comprehending the complexity that lie underlying these reasons. This is like a complex beehive made from the experiences of individual people, medical realities, and the dynamic terrain of cultural standards; it is not just about vanity or societal demands.

Risks and Benefits of Plastic Surgery

The appealing aspect of plastic surgery is frequently found in its capacity for transformation, a change that goes well beyond the physical to affect psychological and emotional spheres. Examining the hazards connected with these operations is necessary to balance the exhilaration with a dose of reality.

Benefits: More Than Skin Deep

Emotional Well-Being

There is a significant psychological boost after a successful treatment. The boost in self-confidence can improve general emotional wellness, from a straightforward rhinoplasty to a complicated reconstructive surgery.

Enhanced Physical Comfort

The comfort and functionality of the body can be greatly increased by procedures like breast reduction or eyelid surgery in addition to offering aesthetic enhancements.

Professional Benefits

As was previously mentioned, visual appeal can be a professional value in several fields.

Health Gains

While not a replacement for leading a healthy lifestyle, some operations, such as liposuction, may help kick-start one.

Societal Reintegration

Reconstructive surgery can provide a path back into society and enable people who have endured tragedy or genetic problems to blend in without being noticed.

Risks: The Other Side of the Coin

Surgical Complications

Surgery always carries some risk. Common dangers to think about include infections, scars, and anesthetic issues.

Financial Strain

Insurance does not typically cover a lot of plastic surgery options, which could be stressful financially.

Psychological Ramifications

Unmet expectations can trigger a variety of mental health problems, such as sadness or body dysmorphia.

Medical Health Concerns

In certain situations, complications can even lead to the development of new health problems or make preexisting ones worse.

Social Stigma

Although cultural acceptance has increased, having plastic surgery still occasionally attracts criticism or censure.

Making informed selections is crucial given the myriad dangers and advantages. Making a well-informed decision can be aided by in-depth consultations with skilled plastic surgeons, live simulations, and recommendations from former clients. Additionally, postoperative care and rigorous following to medical recommendations greatly reduce potential hazards, tilting the balances in favor of a positive outcome.

Cost of Plastic Surgery

When it comes to plastic surgery, the adage "you get what you pay for" is especially applicable. Cutting corners in this area is not advised. The financial commitment, however, extends beyond only the surgeon's price. Here is a full breakdown of the elements that go into the final price.

Professional Fees

Surgeon's Fee

Usually, this fee represents the bulk of the expense. greater levels of experience, specialty, and geographic location typically result in greater fees for surgeons.

Anesthesiologist's Fee

The price of general anesthesia isn't inexpensive, and it often fluctuates depending on how long and involved the treatment is.

Consultation Fees

Initial consultation fees are frequently charged by surgeons and perhaps deducted from the overall cost of the procedure.

Facility Costs

Hospital or Clinic Fees

Additional costs for the surgery itself, as well as any necessary post-op care and overnight stays, may be incurred at the facility where it is performed.

Operating Room Costs

The price of the space itself and any specialist equipment used are also taken into consideration.

Additional Costs

Medical Tests

Costs may increase with pre-operative procedures including blood work, EKGs, or MRIs.

Post-Operative Care

The entire budget should account for additional expenses such as follow-up appointments, specialized clothing, or medical supplies.

Miscellaneous

The whole expense may also be impacted by travel costs, medical costs, and any necessary revision surgeries.

Geographical Variations

Based on the area, costs can vary greatly. Generally speaking, higher surgical expenditures are found in metropolitan locations with higher cost of living.

Payment Plans and Financing

To make operations more affordable, many offices provide a range of payment options. In some cases, financial organizations even provide their own credit schemes or collaborate with other financial institutions.

Insurance Caveats

The majority of cosmetic procedures are regarded as elective and are not consequently protected by insurance. Reconstructive procedures, however, might be funded, at least in part, particularly if they are deemed medically necessary.

When choosing plastic surgery, cost should never be the main consideration, although it undoubtedly plays a big role. Making an informed choice that suits your aesthetic objectives and budgetary capacities can be facilitated by thorough study, consultation with several surgeons, and a well-thought-out budget.

Types of Plastic Surgery Procedures

There is a wide range of plastic surgery treatments, all of which address various needs and preferences. Before selecting an item from the menu, it is necessary to be aware of it.

Facial Procedures

Rhinoplasty

This treatment, also known as a "nose job," alters the nose's size or form.

Blepharoplasty

Sagging or drooping eyelids can be treated by eye bag removal or eyelid surgery.

Facelift

A facelift, also known as a rhytidectomy, tightens the facial muscles and skin for a more youthful appearance.

Body Procedures

Liposuction

This method eliminates surplus fat from particular regions, such as the thighs or abdomen.

Tummy Tuck

This procedure, often known as an abdominoplasty, tightens the abdominal muscles and eliminates excess skin.

Breast Augmentation

In order to enlarge the breasts, this requires the use of implants or fat transfer.

Gender-Specific Procedures

Gynecomastia Surgery

This removes extra breast tissue and is geared toward guys.

Breast Lift

This is specifically designed for women and lifts and tightens the breasts by removing extra skin.

Vaginal Rejuvenation

This category comprises numerous operations to enhance the female genitalia's functionality and appearance.

Reconstructive Procedures

Breast Reconstruction

This usually occurs after a mastectomy and seeks to rebuild a breast that looks natural.

Scar Revision

This employs a number of approaches to reduce the visibility of scars.

Cleft Lip and Palate Repair

Early childhood is usually the time to address this inherent problem.

Minimally Invasive Options

Botox and Fillers

These injectables offer a rapid solution for volume loss and wrinkles.

Chemical Peels

This more superficial treatment exfoliates the skin in order to cure various skin conditions.

PRP Therapy

Due to its rejuvenating effects, platelet-rich plasma is gaining popularity.

Cutting-Edge Procedures

Fat Transfer

This includes shifting fat for contouring or augmentation from one bodily part to another.

Laser Treatments

These are becoming more popular for treating skin conditions and shaving.

3D Imaging

A virtual glimpse of the surgical results is provided by some providers.

To reach the desired result, keep in mind that many of these techniques can be combined or customized. Choosing from a list is less important than working with a skilled surgeon to establish a surgical strategy.

The best course of action for one person could not be the best for another. Before selecting a choice, it is essential to go over your medical background, aesthetic objectives, and lifestyle considerations with your surgeon.

Common Myths About Plastic Surgery

False information spreads quickly in the field of plastic surgery, thus it's critical to separate fact from fiction. Sadly, there are a lot of myths surrounding plastic surgery today due to the growth of social media, dramatic entertainment, and plain ol' gossip. So let's dispel some of the most widely held falsehoods.

#1 Plastic Surgery is Purely Cosmetic

While the cosmetic component frequently garners attention, plastic surgery has a far wider range of applications, including vital reconstructive treatments. We're referring to operations that correct congenital defects, burns, or damage to rehabilitate functionality and aesthetics. In other words, it's not only about looking nice; it's frequently about getting life back to normal.

#2 It's Only for the Wealthy

Despite not being cheap, numerous treatments are now more affordable than ever, thanks in large part to the development of financing solutions. Reconstructive procedures are frequently covered by insurance, too. Therefore, wealth is no longer a rigid bar to this world.

#3 Results Last Forever

'Forever' is pushing it, even if many treatments do provide long-lasting results. While a facelift might turn back the hands of time, it won't stop the process of aging. Your keys to extending those results will be appropriate aftercare, lifestyle decisions, and perhaps touch-up operations.

#4 Recovery is a Walk in the Park

Some people believe they will emerge from the operating room prepared for a red carpet event because of reality television. Reality check: Recovery requires persistence and time. Plan ahead because most surgical procedures involve pain, edema, and recovery time.

#5 It's a 'Vain' Choice

Being confident and at ease in your own flesh is a genuine desire. Procedures provide a path to improved mental health and self-esteem for many people. There is nothing 'vain' about a decision if it has been carefully thought through and appropriate expectations have been set.

#6 Any Doctor Can Do It

Technically, any medical professional is capable of using a scalpel, but would you really want your nose surgery performed by a general practitioner? Years of specialized training are necessary since plastic surgery is both an art and a science. Always seek out board-certified doctors with experience in the particular operation you're thinking about.

#7 It's a Quick Fix for Body Issues

While plastic surgery might alter your face's form or remove years, it cannot replace a healthy way of life. The critical components for long-term success after surgery are weight maintenance, physical activity, and mental health care.

#8 It's Only for Women

Men are visiting plastic surgeons' offices in greater numbers for procedures ranging from body contouring to botox. Plastic surgery is becoming more and more ubiquitous as the societal stigma associated with men and the procedure quickly fades.

#9 It's Only for Older People

Younger people are increasingly choosing prophylactic or minor surgical procedures. Consider "prejuvenation"—taking action before significant aging symptoms manifest.

Plastic surgery is a dynamic discipline that is rife with myths. Your journey will be illuminated by thorough research and advice from qualified experts, who can help you distinguish between enduring truths and transitory misconceptions.

CHAPTER TWO

2. Cosmetic Plastic Surgery for Women

Cosmetic plastic surgery provides a variety of options for ladies who want to improve their outward appearance. There are many alternatives available to address different physical issues, including Brazilian butt lifts, liposuction, stomach tucks, and breast augmentation and lift. In regards to these methods, it's important to distinguish fact from fiction. By accurately describing each procedure's requirements, advantages, and potential disadvantages, this chapter will dispel prevalent misconceptions about cosmetic plastic surgery for women. This chapter will help you choose the best technique for your requirements and preferences, whether you want to increase your self-assurance or are just trying to feel more at ease in your own skin.

Breast Augmentation

Breast augmentation is more than simply a cosmetic change; it's a step in a woman's journey to better self-confidence and wellbeing. Customization is the secret to success in this medical venture.

What is Breast Augmentation?

Let's get the mystery surrounding this common operation out of the way. Breast augmentation is enlarging your breasts by inserting implants or using a fat transfer technique. But it's not just about size. It can offer a more appealing contour, equalize asymmetrical breasts, and replace lost volume from aging or pregnancy.

Implants or Fat Transfer: What's Your Style?

Your unique tastes and medical needs will determine the surgical technique you use.

Implants

These typically have a predetermined form and size and are made of silicone or saline.

Fat Transfer

This is the natural method, in which fat is refined and injected into the breasts from other regions of your body.

Setting Expectations: What Can It Do For You?

Women opt for breast augmentation for a variety of reasons, many of which are particular to themselves and their life stories. There is a customized method for everyone, whether you are a breast cancer survivor seeking post-mastectomy reconstruction or a new mother dissatisfied with post-pregnancy alterations.

Pre-Surgical Preparations: Get Set Go

You'll go through exams including mammograms, consultations, and other procedures to make sure you're a good candidate before the big day. Additionally, during this stage, you and your surgeon go through in great detail your expectations, including implant kind and incision site.

A Closer Look At The Operation

You'll be sedated or under general anesthesia on the day of the procedure. A one- to two-hour time frame is possible for the full process. In order to reduce obvious scarring, your surgeon will make incisions in hidden places before inserting the implants (*Ri et al., 2022*).

Post-Operation: The Recovery Timeline

Recovery goes rather smoothly, however it differs from person to person. You'll start out wearing a special surgical bra, which could be uncomfortable. You can resume your regular activities after a few weeks, but you shouldn't engage in any vigorous exercise until your surgeon gives the all-clear.

Longevity: How Long Do Results Last?

The implants are not lifetime devices, despite the fact that their longevity varies. After 10 to 20 years, depending on the type, you might require a replacement. The integrity of the implants and your health must be maintained through routine examinations.

Breast Lift

Breast lifts, technically referred to as mastopexies, aim to change the position and contour of the breasts, as opposed to breast augmentation, which focuses exclusively on size and volume. Your chest feels as though it has undergone a rebirth, returning you to your more perky youth. What is actually involved, then? Let's go over the specifics.

A breast lift is what?

A surgical technique called a mastopexy is used to lift and reshape drooping breasts. Breast tissue can suffer from the effects of aging, gravity, weight fluctuations, and life events like pregnancy. Your breasts' young posture is restored after a lift, without necessarily changing their size (*Stevens et al., 2007*).

How Does It Differ From Augmentation?

An attempt to increase size or volume is not the goal of a breast lift, despite common belief. In order to lift the breast, the skin around it must be tightened, the nipple and areola must be relocated, and sometimes superfluous tissue must be removed.

To Lift or Not to Lift: Are You a Candidate?

What criteria do you use to determine whether a breast lift is the right procedure for you? Your indications to think about this procedure include sagging or drooping breasts, stretched skin, and a flattened breast shape. A breast lift may be especially helpful for women who have recently had pregnancy, breastfeeding, or a large reduction of weight.

The Method Behind the Magic: Surgical Techniques

Depending on the quantity of excess skin, the existing breast tissue, and your individual goals, your surgeon may employ one of a number of procedures. Circular incisions around the areola, keyhole cuts, and inverted T-shapes are typical incision designs. Your surgeon will assist you in selecting the approach that is best for you because each has advantages and disadvantages.

Recovery and Aftercare

You will cover gauze dressings with an elastic bandage or surgical bra after surgery. To drain any extra blood or fluid, a little tube may also be inserted just under the skin. You should expect a two-week recuperation period right away, but over the following six weeks, you should gradually resume your normal activities.

A breast lift produces quick effects, but there is a catch, as with everything good. Although the surgery cannot reverse the effects of time, you can extend the life of your results by avoiding unhealthy habits and keeping your weight constant.

Liposuction

Let's dispel the mystery. The undesired fat deposits in some parts of the body can be removed through a surgical treatment called liposuction. This results in a physique that is more defined and well-balanced. Not losing weight is the major objective here; rather, sculpting and reshaping the body is the focus.

The Science and the Art: Techniques Involved

The procedures have progressed from the traditional suction-assisted liposuction to the more sophisticated laser-assisted variants of the procedure. But in the end, they all accomplish the same objective, which is to break down fat and remove it. Some of the approaches involve the use of high-frequency vibrations, while others involve the use of laser beams, and yet others involve the use of water jets. The option that is best for you will be determined by the kind of fat you have and where it is located (*A Journey Through Liposuction and Liposculture: Review, 2017*).

Me, Myself, and Lipo: Who Needs It?

Those who have stubborn fat deposits in specific areas of the body that cannot be reduced by diet and exercise are good candidates for liposuction. However, this is not a method that can be applied universally. The selection process takes into consideration factors like as your overall health, the suppleness of your skin, and the kind of expectations you have for the procedure. If you're looking for a fast way to lose weight and are considering liposuction as an option, you should reconsider. It's more of a finishing touch than a beginning point, if that makes any sense.

Price Tag and Piggy Banks: What Will It Cost?

Cheaper isn't better when it comes to medical procedures, despite the fact that it can be tempting to look for deals. You should plan on spending between $2,000 and $3,500 for each treatment area, on average. This pricing does not include any additional charges such as those for anesthesia, the facilities in the operating room, or any other expenditures associated with the procedure.

Post-Surgery and Peace

Recovery time may be short, but you shouldn't instantly sign up for a marathon after you've had surgery. Initial symptoms typically consist of bruising, pain, and swelling. Compression clothing is your new best buddy because it helps reduce swelling and improves contour. The majority of people are able to return to work within a few days to a week, although they should refrain from engaging in physically taxing activities for around one month.

The benefits of liposuction are permanent as long as the patient continues to maintain a healthy weight and an active lifestyle. But keep in mind that things outside of your control, such as the effects of natural aging or weight increase, can influence the outcomes. It's possible that you'll need periodic touch-ups in order to keep your optimum form.

Tummy Tuck

Abdominoplasty, also referred to as a stomach tuck in the medical community, is not merely a temporary treatment for abdominal fat. Instead, it's a surgical technique designed to make the abdomen more solid and smooth by pulling together any weak or divided muscles. When food and exercise fall short in toning this key area of the body, this is the solution of choice.

Choosing Your Path: Types of Tummy Tucks

Yes, there are options available, even for belly tucks. The total abdominoplasty is a good option for people who require considerable treatment. It entails making an incision that extends from the navel to the lower abdomen. For patients who just require skin removal from below the navel, mini-abdominoplasties are available. Another option is an extended stomach tuck, which also corrects the flanks and sides.

Am I the One? Identifying Candidates

The procedure known as an abdominoplasty is mainly for people who have previously dropped a large amount of weight but still have extra skin and fat (Regan & Casaubon, 2023). Additionally, it is well-liked by women who have had several pregnancies. This might not be the best moment for the operation if you're anticipating future pregnancies or major weight loss.

Investing in You: Let's Talk Money

The price of a belly tuck varies depending on a number of variables, such as where you live, how skilled the surgeon is, and how complicated the procedure is. Budget carefully because most health insurance plans do not cover cosmetic treatments, so be prepared to spend anywhere between $3,000 and $12,000.

The Aftermath: Recovery and What to Expect

Some downtime is expected. Your abdominal area will be patched and wrapped as soon as the surgical procedure is complete. For around six weeks, you might need to support your abdomen and reduce swelling by using a compression garment. Especially if you have young children, getting back to normal can take a few weeks, so make sure you have some help around the house.

The Unveiling: Long-term Results and Upkeep

Your new stomach will be obvious right away, but the full effects won't be seen until the swelling goes down. Keep up a healthy diet and consistent workout routine for long-term results. Maintaining a constant weight is essential because significant weight changes might negatively impact your outcomes.

Brazilian Butt Lift (BBL)

More than just a passing fad, the Brazilian Butt Lift (or BBL) allows you to make the most of your own body fat to enhance and reshape your buttocks' natural curves. Yes, you heard correctly. Instead of a man-made implant, your fat takes center stage.

The Core Principle: Fat Transfer

The buttocks fat is transferred from other areas of the body (usually the belly, thighs, or back) via liposuction and then injected. Your rear end will look bigger and more young as a result of improving the volume and form. The risk of issues that can occur from synthetic materials is decreased by using your own fat *("Brazilian Butt Lift" Performed by Board-Certified Brazilian Plastic Surgeons: Reports of an Expert Opinion Survey - PubMed, 2019).*

To BBL or Not to BBL: Ideal Candidates

Are you unsure of your suitability as a candidate? Those who desire to enhance their buttocks' size and attractiveness but already have sufficient fat reserves elsewhere in their bodies are the greatest candidates for this surgery. It is more than just a vanity play; by addressing inequalities and asymmetries, it can also be useful.

What Will It Cost?

Brazilian butt lift prices fluctuate according to factors such as the quality of the surgeon, the amount of the procedure, and the patient's geographic location. Typically, the price range is between $4,000 and $15,000. Insurance won't cover the cost because it's a cosmetic procedure, so be sure your funds are in order.

Charting the Road to Recovery

For around two weeks following the procedure, you will need to avoid sitting directly on your buttocks, which requires you to spend most of the time either on your stomach or upright. A BBL is not for the weak of heart, even if it will be uncomfortable. Although recovery takes time, the majority of people may resume their regular activities within a month and go back to work within 2-3 weeks.

Playing the Long Game: Sustaining the Results

A BBL's joy comes from its long-lasting effects. The transferred fat cells are permanent once they are in place. However, a substantial weight gain or loss can change your results. The best way to prolong the pleasure of your new curves is to stick to a balanced diet and keep a steady weight through regular exercise.

The Brazilian Butt Lift is a natural method of butt augmentation, but it also carries some risks. The treatment requires a substantial commitment, from picking the best physician to adhering to thorough aftercare.

Facelift

We frequently remark that age is simply a number, yet our skin rarely hears this. A facelift might be the best option to consider if you're hoping for more dramatic results than what creams other non-surgical procedures can provide. Let's explore the purpose of this surgery and the potential beneficiaries.

A Facelift in a Nutshell

"Rhytidectomy," the surgical operation that tightens and eliminates drooping skin on the face and neck, is the medical word for a facelift. In a sense, it's a skin makeover that aims to get rid of wrinkles, deep creases, and loose skin—all telltale indicators of age (*Sanan & Most, 2021*).

Differences From Non-Surgical Treatments

A facelift is comprehensive as opposed to Botox or fillers, which focus on particular problem areas. It deals with the neck as well as the lower two-thirds of your face. It also involves a lengthier recuperation period, but the results are more profound and long-lasting as a result.

Who Makes the Cut? Ideal Clients

When considering whether or not to get a facelift, it's important to think about things like your skin's elasticity, your bone structure, and your general health. Candidates typically have considerable face sagging but have some degree of skin elasticity. It's not just an option for those in their golden years; many people in their forties and fifties also seek out anti-aging procedures.

Price Tag: What's the Damage?

A facelift is not inexpensive. You should expect to pay anywhere from $7,000 and $15,000, depending on the complexity of the procedure and the surgeon's experience. It's a large financial commitment, so it's essential to know what you need and what you want.

Navigating the Aftermath: Recovery

You can anticipate wearing bandages and perhaps some drainage tubes after surgery. In addition to swelling, bruising, and the need to stay out of the sun for a while, recovery can take several weeks. These post-operative annoyances eventually disappear, revealing your refreshed appearance.

Maintaining Your Youth: Longevity of Results

Depending on how carefully you take care of your skin following surgery, the results of a facelift can last up to 10 years. In order to preserve the results, this entails a rigorous skincare routine and maybe further non-surgical procedures like fillers or Botox.

Even while a facelift gives the illusion of being more youthful, it is not a permanent fix for aging. It necessitates dedication to the treatment as well as the follow-up care. Therefore, a facelift may be the best option if you want to make a lasting investment in your physical appearance.

Rhinoplasty

Rhinoplasty, also referred to as a "nose job," is much more than just a cosmetic procedure. Even though it's a very common cosmetic operation, its reach also includes practical problems like breathing difficulties.

What is a rhinoplasty exactly?

Rhinoplasty, to put it simply, is the surgical remodeling of the nose. Whether you have a bulge on your nose's bridge, wide nostrils, or an awkward angle where your nose meets your upper lip, rhinoplasty can help. If you have a deviated septum or another structural condition that's affecting your breathing, this treatment option can help.

Distinguishing Cosmetic and Functional Rhinoplasty

The goal of aesthetic rhinoplasty is to modify the nose's size and form in order to better balance face proportions. On the other hand, functional rhinoplasty aims to address problems that impede breathing or lead to persistent congestion. Many people choose to combine the two, boosting the nose's appearance and functionality (*Zhu et al., 2022*).

Who's In? Ideal Candidates for Rhinoplasty

Those who are dissatisfied with the way their nose looks or who have functional problems that traditional procedures have failed to remedy are good candidates. Age is a factor as well; it is advised to postpone the treatment until the nose has grown to its mature size, usually around the age of 16.

How Deep is the Dent in Your Wallet?

Rhinoplasty is not an inexpensive procedure. Aesthetic rhinoplasty is typically not covered by medical insurance, and the associated expenses can range anywhere from $5,000 to $15,000, depending on a number of factors such as the level of experience of the surgeon and the geographic area. Insurance companies may provide coverage for functional rhinoplasty, which aims to address breathing problems.

The Path to Your New Nose: Surgical Procedures

There are many different surgical methods, but the majority of them entail creating incisions inside the nostrils to gain access to the bones and cartilage. The interior structures are then reshaped by surgeons to get the desired appearance. General or local anesthesia may be utilized during the procedure, which normally lasts one to two hours.

Healing and Aftercare: The Long Road to Recovery

Weeks-long recovery processes necessitate lots of rest and minimal exercise. Initial bruising and swelling are frequent, but these eventually go away. During the first stage of healing, a splint or packing material may be applied to aid in maintaining the new shape.

Although rhinoplasty has both functional and aesthetic advantages, it's necessary to have realistic expectations. Not perfection but improvement is the aim. It is crucial to have a full consultation with your surgeon to go over your goals and potential outcomes.

Eyelid Surgery

No matter how energized you feel, have you ever had the impression that the mirror shows an older, worn-out version of yourself? Undereye bags or drooping eyelids that betray your vitality may be the only culprit. This situation calls for blepharoplasty, sometimes known as eyelid surgery.

What is Eyelid Surgery?

Through surgery called blepharoplasty, flaws around the eyes can be improved by removing or relocating extra skin, muscle, and even fat. The procedure can restore youthful curves, whether you have sagging upper lids or big bags under your eyes.

Upper Eyelid vs Lower Eyelid Surgery

Upper and lower eyelid surgery are the two categories into which the procedure can be divided. The upper variety removes extra skin that obstructs vision or is unsightly. The main reasons for lower eyelid surgery are to get rid of bags under the eyes and lessen wrinkles (*Naik et al., 2009*).

Who Should Consider Eyelid Surgery?

Blepharoplasty could be the game-changer you're looking for if you struggle with blurry vision caused by sagging upper lids or believe that bags under your eyes give you a perpetually exhausted appearance. Adults over the age of 35 are the target audience for the treatment, however younger people with severe eyelid issues may also choose to have it done.

Is Your Wallet Ready?

The costs can be rather high, in the range of $2,000-$5,000 depending on the quality of the surgeon and the patient's location, just like with any other elective cosmetic treatment. Unless the operation is medically necessary to improve vision, insurance is typically not an option because it is frequently regarded as cosmetic.

Procedure Specifics: What to Expect

The procedure typically lasts between one and two hours and is normally done while sedated and under local anaesthetic. To reduce obvious scarring, incisions are done along the natural contours of the eyes. The extra skin and fat are subsequently eliminated or realigned, and the wounds are then stitched or sealed with skin adhesive.

After the Cuts: Recovery Insights

Expect some swelling, bruising, and discomfort following surgery. These symptoms can be treated with elevation and cold compresses. After around 10 days, the majority of people can resume their regular activities, however individual recovery times do vary. For best outcomes, it's essential to adhere to your surgeon's post-operative instructions.

Although eyelid surgery provides long-lasting improvements, it cannot reverse the effects of aging. Even though blepharoplasty will always make your eyes appear younger than they would have otherwise, your eyes will still continue to age naturally. Maintenance operations, such as brow lifts and filler injections, might further improve your appearance if you're serious about keeping your results.

With eyelid surgery, you should look more rested, with wide eyes that reflect your true spirit. Given its transforming power, it should come as no surprise that blepharoplasty has drawn the interest of those looking to rejuvenate and brighten their eyes.

Lip Augmentation

Sometimes, the naturally larger, more sensuous lips we desire don't exactly match the lips we are born with. An aesthetic surgery called lip augmentation uses a variety of methods, from surgical implants to injectable fillers, to give you the larger, more balanced lips you've always wanted.

What is Lip Augmentation?

A cosmetic treatment called lip augmentation can give you larger, plumper lips. Nowadays, the most popular technique is an injectable dermal filler. These fillers have ingredients that give your lips more volume.

Types of Lip Fillers

Although there are many other types of fillers on the market, hyaluronic acid-based fillers have become more common because of their safer and more natural results. Although they are less frequently performed today, additional forms include lip implants, collagen, and fat injections.

Are You a Good Fit for Lip Augmentation?

You might be a good candidate if you want more volume, a more symmetrical lip shape, or even a younger look. You might have to forego this operation if you currently have cold sores, diabetes, or lupus (*Lip Augmentation: Background, History of the Procedure, Problem, 2023*).

What's the Price Point?

Depending on the method you choose and the location where it is performed, lip augmentation costs can vary. Between $500 to $2,000 can be spent on hyaluronic acid fillers, whereas $5,000 can be spent on surgery.

The Procedure: An Overview

The method for non-surgical procedures is rather straightforward. The lips are first given a numbing agent. After that, the filler is injected into the desired locations. It takes between 15 and 60 minutes to complete the process. Small incisions are made in the corners of the mouth during surgical options, and synthetic or biological materials are then placed.

Recovery and Longevity: What Comes After

Common post-procedure adverse effects include mild swelling and bruising, which usually go away after a week. Around six months following the initial application of fillers, the treatment can be repeated. Surgical methods present longer-lasting fixes but also carry higher hazards.

The End Game: Managing Expectations

The outcomes are often excellent but not shocking. It's important to control your expectations and choose a natural look because too much filler might result in what are referred to as "duck lips."

All in all, lip augmentation presents a fascinating way to improve your facial appearance. A plumper lip can just be a doctor's appointment away, whether you opt for a transient filler or a longer-lasting surgical surgery. As with any elective cosmetic operation, it's important to do your research and talk to your doctor about your options.

Cheek Augmentation

The cosmetic treatment known as cheek augmentation seeks to make your cheeks look younger and more prominent. This procedure offers a number of ways to increase volume to your cheek area, from injectable fillers to surgical implants.

What Exactly is Cheek Augmentation?

The goal of the surgery is to elevate or add volume to the cheek area by focusing on the soft tissue beneath the cheekbones. Your facial contour can be redefined and reshaped, giving you the desired youthful appearance or prominent cheekbones.

Surgical vs. Non-Surgical: Choices Abound

You have choices when it comes to approaches. A more long-lasting option is surgical cheek implants, which include placing a silicone implant above the cheekbones. Dermal fillers, however, provide a less intrusive, albeit short-term, option.

Are You a Candidate for Cheek Augmentation?

You can be a good candidate if you want more facial definition and have hollow or flat cheeks. Aging-related face volume loss may also be helped. However, people who have specific medical conditions or are taking particular drugs might not be eligible (*Sadick & Palmisano, 2009*).

What's the Damage?

Depending on the filler and the required volume, dermal fillers can cost anywhere from $600 to $3,000 each treatment. On the other hand, surgical implants might cost anywhere from $2,000 and $10,000, depending on the surgeon's fees and the patient's location.

The Procedure Unveiled

A little incision is made inside the mouth or along the hairline for surgical procedures. After that, an implant is positioned above or below the cheekbone. Filler material is injected with a syringe into specific locations on the cheek in the case of fillers. Both operations could use sedatives or a local anesthetic.

Post-Procedure

For surgical treatments, you can anticipate a two-week recuperation period during which you'll feel some swelling and soreness. The downtime for fillers is minimal, however slight swelling and bruising are common.

Maintaining the Look

Depending on the filler used, effects may gradually wane over a period of 6 to 24 months, necessitating retouching. Surgical implants provide a more long-lasting result, but even they can't stop the aging process entirely.

Results: Keep it Realistic

Although having your cheeks augmented can greatly improve your appearance, you and your physician should be on the same page regarding the procedure's risks and benefits. Balance is important since over-augmentation might result in an artificial, "puffy" appearance.

There are several ways to improve your facial profile with cheek augmentation, and selecting the best one for you requires a thorough consultation with a licensed medical specialist. You may choose the finest option for your aesthetic journey by being informed about every aspect of any cosmetic surgery.

Botox and Fillers

Botox and fillers are the undisputed king and queen of non-invasive cosmetic procedures. However, what exactly are they, how do they vary, and what benefits do they provide? Without any further ado, let's begin.

The wrinkle whisperer, Botox

The bacterium Clostridium botulinum is the source of the injectable neurotoxin known as Botox. What makes it famous? creases can be minimized by briefly paralyzing muscles. It primarily targets forehead wrinkles, frown lines, and crow's feet (*Fink & Prager, 2014*) .

Fillers: The Volume Vendors

Dermal fillers, as opposed to Botox, which inhibits muscle activation, concentrate on increasing tissue volume. Lips and cheeks, for example, can have their volume restored using these products, which are typically produced from hyaluronic acid. They provide a kind of quick facelift without undergoing surgery.

Pick Your Potion: Botox or Fillers?

Botox is the solution if you're worried about lines that show when you scowl, frown, or look puzzled. Fillers, on the other hand, will probably be your first choice if sagging or volume loss keeps you up at night. To gain from both, many people choose to combine them.

Cost Comparison: What's the Dent in the Wallet?

Each unit of botox typically costs $10 to $20, and 20 to 60 units are needed for a single treatment. But the cost of fillers is determined by the number and type required; prices per syringe range from $600 to $2,000.

Procedure Particulars

Both treatments are completed in between 15 and 60 minutes. While fillers may need slightly larger needles or even microcannulas, botox takes a succession of tiny injections with a fine needle. For comfort, numbing cream or local anesthetic are frequently used.

Recovery and Risks: Short and Sweet

You can resume most activities right away after Botox and fillers, both of which have a short recovery period. A little bruising or swelling is typical. The outcomes could be uneven, there could be minimal scarring, and in rare instances, there could be allergic responses.

Longevity of Results: Temporary but Repeatable

Follow-up sessions are necessary to maintain results because Botox typically lasts three to six months. Depending on the type and location treated, fillers can last anywhere from six months to two years.

The Right Provider: Your Aesthetic Ally

There are many providers due to the popularity of these therapies, but not all of them are the same. Choose a dermatologist or plastic surgeon with board certification who has knowledge with injectables.

Botox and fillers provide effective alternatives to surgery for face rejuvenation. Although they target different problems—Botox reduces dynamic wrinkles, while fillers increase volume—they frequently function as complementing treatments in an all-encompassing anti-aging plan. The secret is to speak with a qualified expert to develop a personalized treatment plan that fits your cosmetic objectives.

Laser Treatments

Beyond the world of science fiction, laser procedures have made a significant impact on aesthetic medicine. They have emerged as the preferred method for treating a variety of skin issues, from obstinate scars to unwanted hair.

The ABCs of Lasers

We refer to Light Amplification by Stimulated Emission of Radiation (laser) when we use the term. In simple terms? controlled light beams with different levels of skin penetration. To choose the most suitable laser type for you, it is essential to speak with an expert practitioner because each laser type is tailored for particular treatments.

Different Lasers, Different Gains

The diversity is remarkable, ranging from ablative lasers that remove the top layers of skin to non-ablative lasers that heat the underlying skin tissue without causing damage to the surface. Erbium lasers, fractional lasers, and CO_2 lasers are examples of common types. Each has a different area of expertise, such as skin resurfacing, scar minimization, or hair removal (*Khalkhal et al., 2019*).

Cost and Commitment

The cost of a laser treatment typically ranges from $200 to $3,000 each session. Depending on the type of treatment and each person's needs, different sessions may be required. Budget for the entire treatment cycle because cosmetic operations are typically not covered by health insurance.

The Procedure and What to Expect

Depending on the treatment region, a typical session can last anywhere from 20 minutes to an hour. An ice pack or local anesthetic will be used to numb your skin before the procedure begins. As the laser works, you can experience what seems like a rubber band cracking against your skin.

Short-Term and Long-Term Effects

Your skin will probably be red and puffy right after treatment, feeling somewhat like a slight sunburn. Long-term effects are possible, however maintenance sessions are frequently advised. Consider the removal of acne scars as an example; to maintain the softer skin texture, periodic follow-up treatments may be necessary.

Safety and Potential Side Effects

While typically risk-free when carried out by trained experts, laser treatments do have some downsides. Burns, scars, and variations in skin color are a few examples of these. These hazards and ways to reduce them should be thoroughly covered at your pre-treatment consultation.

Aftercare is a Must

After treatment, you'll need to be vigilant about sun protection. You might also be given prescriptions for specialized skincare items to speed up recovery. The risk of problems is increased and results may be compromised if aftercare is neglected.

The end result is that laser skin resurfacing offers a very flexible method of skin enhancement. Lasers are a less invasive option that frequently yields impressive results, whether you're trying to reduce scars, get rid of hair, or get a younger-looking skin. However, appropriate advice and expert execution are the keys to success, so be sure to put time and effort into choosing your practitioner.

CHAPTER THREE

3. Reconstructive Plastic Surgery for Women

Plastic surgery can be a crucial tool for rebuilding and healing the body after trauma or illness, in addition to improving one's looks. Reconstructive plastic surgery can provide women who have undergone cancer treatment, been injured, or have birth abnormalities with hope and recovery. This chapter will discuss the many reconstructive techniques that are available to women, such as tissue expander treatments, scar revision, burn reconstruction, cleft lip and palate repair, and breast reconstruction. We'll discuss the difficulties faced by women who have had these surgeries as well as strategies for helping them reclaim their self-worth. By focusing light on these frequently disregarded practices, we seek to encourage hope and resiliency in people who might be dealing with same difficulties.

Breast Reconstruction

After a mastectomy for breast cancer, the road to breast reconstruction is frequently rocky. It's not simply for show; it's a very personal decision made with the intention of regaining not just shape but also a sense of identity and wholeness.

The Rundown on Breast Reconstruction

Breast reconstruction aims to recreate the breast mound in order to match its counterpart's size, shape, and contour. It is possible to use synthetic implants or tissue taken from another area of the body, such as the back or abdomen. Sometimes combining the two yields the most organic outcome.

Timing is Everything: Immediate vs. Delayed

Immediate reconstruction follows a mastectomy, whereas delayed reconstruction is performed after the patient has healed and, in many cases, finished other therapies including chemotherapy and radiation. It is imperative that you and your medical team discuss scheduling because each choice has advantages and disadvantages.

The Surgical Playbook: Techniques Explored

An "flap" of tissue from another area of the body is used in autologous tissue repair. Implant-based reconstruction, on the other hand, makes use of silicone or saline gel implants. Direct-to-implant reconstruction is a more recent technique that enables the implantation of a permanent implant right away following a mastectomy, frequently with outstanding cosmetic results (*Somogyi et al., 2018*).

Insurance and Costs: The Financial Side

Insurance providers are required to pay for breast reconstruction following a mastectomy in many nations. However, the extent of coverage may vary, so be prepared with all the information. Costs can fluctuate widely depending on factors including the degree of difficulty and whether or not other treatments, such as nipple rebuilding or contralateral balancing procedures, are required.

The Recovery Roadmap

After the procedure, you'll probably spend a few days in the hospital before recovering at home for many weeks. A healthy drug regimen can help you cope with common symptoms including pain, swelling, and exhaustion. It can take 6 to 8 weeks to resume regular activity.

Longevity and Maintenance: What Comes Next?

Although the effects of breast reconstruction are intended to last a lifetime, some procedures, particularly implant-based reconstruction, may need to be redone in the future. In addition, regular mammograms and oncological treatment after a cancer diagnosis are crucial.

Soul Food: Emotional and Psychological Impact

The process frequently has a significant negative effect on mental health and self-esteem. Psychological support is a crucial component of holistic treatment because it is usual to feel a variety of emotions, from relief to grief.

Successful breast reconstruction planning demands candid discussions with your healthcare experts, careful consideration of your options, and an in-depth awareness of your unique physical and emotional requirements. Even though the journey may be challenging, many people view it as a positive experience that improves their physical and spiritual well-being.

Cleft Lip and Palate Repair

Beyond just cosmetics, practical advancements that can dramatically improve quality of life are at the heart of the cleft lip and palate repair tale. Openings in the top lip and/or the roof of the mouth are characteristics of the congenital diseases known as cleft lip and palate. In order to provide an easier transition to normal speech and eating, the treatment aims to shut these holes.

The Fundamentals: What is Cleft Lip and Palate Repair?

Repairing a cleft lip or palate is complex surgery that involves stitching together the lip and/or the roof of the mouth. This normally entails a number of treatments, starting commonly in infancy and frequently continuing until adolescence.

Types of Clefts and their Classification

Lips, palates, or both may develop clefts that are unilateral (on one side only) or bilateral (on both sides). Understanding the nature and size of the cleft informs the surgical technique chosen and affects the order in which the procedure(s) are performed.

Treatment Stages: A Phased Approach

The infant often has their first cleft lip repair surgery between the ages of 3 and 6 months. Palate healing often follows at between six and twelve months. As the kid develops, additional procedures can be required, frequently to enhance speech or the position of the teeth (*Plastic Surgery for Cleft Palate: Cleft Palate, Cleft Palate Appearance, How Does Cleft Palate Affect Hearing and Speech?, 2019*).

Surgical Techniques and Innovations

The Millard approach for cleft lip correction and other types of palatoplasty are two of the surgical methods that can be used. Both functional and aesthetically pleasing results have been enhanced by improvements in surgical techniques, such as the use of endoscopic approaches.

Impact on Feeding and Speech

The effect of cleft repair on speech and nutrition is among its most important features. A child's ability to eat and speak normally can be significantly improved by effective repair, while speech therapy is frequently advised to maximize outcomes.

Financial and Insurance Considerations

It's important to note that because cleft lip and palate correction is regarded as a medically required procedure, the majority of health insurance policies cover it. Do your research because the coverage may vary and out-of-pocket expenses may be high.

Emotional and Psychological Bearings

The psychological and emotional effects of cleft healing are incalculable. Following surgery, children frequently feel an increase in self-esteem and confidence, which has a domino effect on their social relationships and academic achievement.

Long-Term Outlook and Care

Most children who have their cleft lips and/or palates repaired go on to enjoy healthy, productive lives, although they often require additional care, such as dental and/or orthodontic treatments, for the rest of their lives.

Cleft lip and palate repair is a revolutionary set of treatments that can significantly improve a child's capacity for regular breathing, eating, and speaking while also enhancing facial beauty. Even while it requires a lengthy commitment, the numerous advantages make it a game-changing decision for many families.

Scar Revision

Revision of scars has purposes beyond aesthetics. Scars may frequently be a physical and mental burden, impacting not only how you look but also how you feel about yourself. Additionally, some scars may restrict functionality and range of motion. The goal of scar revision surgery is to reduce the scar and, if necessary, restore function while also blending it more smoothly with the surrounding skin tone and texture.

What is Scar Revision?

Scar revision, to put it simply, is a surgical procedure performed to change the appearance of scar tissue with the ultimate goal of lessening its visibility or improving mobility. It's not just for show; a strategically placed surgical procedure can significantly improve your quality of life.

Types of Scars and Their Complexity

Hypertrophic, keloidal, contracture, and acne scars are only a few of the several types of scars that exist. Each has its own characteristics and difficulties. For instance, keloids grow past the original wound's border while hypertrophic scars are red and elevated but typically remain within it. After a burn, contractures frequently develop and limit motion. For a revision to be successful, it is important to identify the type of scar.

Surgical Procedures: A Toolbox of Techniques

The surgical strategy mostly depends on the kind of scar. Options include tissue expansion, dermabrasion, Z-plasty and its variants, laser surgery, and dermabrasion. The choice is frequently influenced by the scar's location, type, and patient's skin condition. Each procedure has advantages and disadvantages (*Ogawa, 2019*).

Risks and Considerations

Despite the potential benefits of scar modification, there are dangers involved, including anesthetic difficulties and infection. The surgeon's expertise is crucial because the surgery calls for a unique set of approaches to produce the best results. Make sure you are therefore in competent hands.

Post-Surgery: The Recovery Timeline

Depending on the operation and the person's general condition, recovery varies. After surgery, topical treatments could help the scar look better. It's typical to experience some redness and swelling, which eventually go away.

Insurance and Cost Factors

Scar revision is frequently not covered by insurance companies because they view it as elective and cosmetic. However, there may be justification for partial or full coverage if the scar is interfering with functionality. Always check with your insurance company and obtain a precise cost estimate in advance.

Emotional and Psychological Impacts

Beyond the outward modifications, reducing a scar successfully might bring about significant emotional relief. It frequently results in greater self-assurance and an enhanced sense of general wellbeing.

The Long-term Prognosis

No scar can actually be fully eliminated. Not perfection but improvement is the goal. The degree to which post-operative care instructions, such as sun protection and the application of topical medications as instructed, are rigorously followed also affects the outcome.

Scar revision provides a chance to lessen the cosmetic and practical effects of scarring, but having reasonable expectations is essential. The advantages can be maximized both physically and psychologically by selecting a trained surgeon and according to pre- and post-operative instructions.

Burn Reconstruction

Burns do more than only leave visible scars. They may cause a wide range of issues, from impaired mobility to psychological harm. Thankfully, improvements in reconstructive surgery have created fresh opportunities for improved results.

What is Burn Reconstruction?

A surgical treatment called burn reconstruction aims to improve the appearance and function of burn-affected areas. Not only are cosmetic details involved; we're also talking about restoring muscle, bone, and skin layers.

Classification of Burns

The key to treating a burn is to comprehend its severity. While first-degree burns typically heal without surgery, second-degree burns may necessitate skin grafts. Deeper tissue destruction is a common occurrence in third- and fourth-degree burns, necessitating more difficult reconstructive treatments.

The Stages of Reconstruction

The primary goals of initial therapies are wound care and infection control. Reconstructive procedures like skin grafts, tissue expansion, and free flap surgeries frequently start weeks or even months after the initial procedure. Multiple surgeries over the course of years may be necessary in cases of severe deformity or functional impairment (*Barret, 2004*).

Skin Grafts and Beyond

Utilizing healthy skin from another region of the body, skin transplants are the most popular procedure. More severe cases can call either tissue expansion procedures or artificial skin procedures, which extend the skin by inserting balloons beneath it. Each method has a unique set of benefits and drawbacks that will be catered to your particular circumstances.

Risks and Challenges

Like every surgical operation, burn reconstruction carries a unique set of hazards, such as those related to anesthesia, infection, and graft failure. Additionally, because burn scars are so complicated, the surgical result might not be as predictable as with other kinds of reconstructive surgery.

Finances and Insurance

Burn reconstruction is frequently deemed medically necessary, resulting in insurance coverage that may be partial or complete, while cosmetic surgeries are typically not covered by insurance. To prevent unforeseen costs, it is advisable to review the specifications of your plan in advance.

The Emotional Angle

It's important to remember that severe burns might result in psychological damage. Successful burn reconstruction has the ability to change lives on a far deeper level than just the surface, frequently serving as a catalyst for longer-lasting emotional and psychological recovery.

Long-term Outlook

After surgery, continued treatment may include physical therapy, therapies for managing scars, and follow-up appointments at regular intervals to assess how well the reconstruction is holding up. To further improve the treated area's appearance and functionality, more treatments may be scheduled.

Recovery from a burn injury is a complex process that necessitates not only medical know-how but also a comprehensive strategy that takes into account the patient's mental and emotional well-being. The aim is to heal more than just your skin so that you may lead a regular life again.

Vaginal Rejuvenation

Concerns that affect a woman's quality of life are receiving increasing attention as discussions about women's health become less taboo. Vaginal health is one of them, particularly after childbirth, during menopause, or as we age naturally. A range of operations aiming at enhancing both function and beauty in this private area are included under the umbrella term of "vaginal rejuvenation."

What Exactly is Vaginal Rejuvenation?

Contrary to popular belief, vaginal rejuvenation has more benefits than only cosmetics. Incontinence, vaginal laxity, and dryness are just a few of the issues that can be addressed surgically or non-surgically. There are various options, including laser procedures and labiaplasty, to suit different demands.

Who Can Benefit?

The choice to have vaginal rejuvenation is highly individual. Women who have laxity that reduces sexual satisfaction, have incontinence, or have discomfort from large labia are the best prospects. The hormonal changes brought on by menopause and childbirth also contribute to the modifications that can be treated by these procedures.

Understanding the Procedures

The two most popular surgical procedures are vaginoplasty and labiaplasty. Vaginoplasty tightens the vaginal canal while labiaplasty cuts extra tissue from the labia for a more symmetrical appearance. In order to achieve a natural tightening effect, non-surgical methods including laser and radiofrequency treatments encourage collagen formation (*Barbara et al., 2017*).

The Crucial Role of Consultation

Just the beginning involves selecting a skilled surgeon. A thorough consultation where you may go through your issues, goals, and medical background ensures that the treatment plan is personalized for you. Make careful to inquire about the expected outcomes, dangers, and recuperation time.

Risks and Side Effects

Risks associated with infection or scarring exist with every surgical procedure. Although generally less harmful, non-surgical treatments might nonetheless cause short-term discomfort or sensory alterations. These dangers can be reduced with thorough preoperative tests and conversations.

A Word on Finances

These operations are typically paid for out-of-pocket because insurance companies frequently classify them as aesthetic rather than medically required. Geographical location and the particular operation undergone can affect pricing.

Emotional and Psychological Impact

In addition to the physical benefits, vaginal rejuvenation frequently improves self-esteem and rekindles close relationships. Following surgery, many women report improved sexual experiences, which improves emotional wellbeing in general.

Aftercare and Longevity

The importance of aftercare cannot be overstated, whether you choose surgery or non-surgical treatment. The outcome of the treatment will depend on how well you heed the surgeon's instructions regarding resumed sexual activity, physical activity, and other activities.

Not merely a trendy term, vaginal rejuvenation is a growing area of plastic surgery that holistically improves a woman's quality of life. This is about encouraging women to live comfortably and confidently, not about submitting to social expectations.

Tissue Expander Procedures

Tissue expanders frequently serve a crucial role in the field of reconstructive plastic surgery, enabling doctors to basically "create" more skin for use in mending or reconstructing different body parts. When substantial areas of skin are missing or injured, as after a mastectomy, from serious burns, or from traumatic injuries, they can completely modify the situation.

The 'What' of Tissue Expanders

A medically inserted silicone balloon-like tool called a tissue expander is gradually inflated over time after being surgically put beneath the skin. This gradually stretches the nearby tissue, encouraging the creation of new skin. After that, the fresh skin might be used during other reconstructive treatments.

How Does It Work?

A saline solution is gradually added to the tissue expander after it has been subcutaneously implanted during the initial surgery over the course of a few weeks or months. The method for accomplishing this is a tiny valve that is either a part of the expander or is positioned beneath the skin. These routine "fill-ups" lead the expander to swell, progressively expanding the surrounding skin (*Tzolova & Hadjiiski, 2008*).

Who's a Candidate?

The majority of patients who need considerable skin repair but lack sufficient nearby tissue for grafting are good candidates for tissue expander treatments. They're frequently utilized in pediatric plastic surgery for issues like congenital nevi (large birthmarks), but they're also frequently employed in breast reconstruction after mastectomy.

Procedure Techniques

There are frequently two steps to the process. In the first, the expander is inserted; in the second, it is taken out and the new skin is used for reconstruction. The expander may occasionally be used with an acellular dermal matrix to increase support and enhance the ultimate aesthetic outcome.

Risks and Complications

The danger of tissue enlargement is the same as it is with any surgical operation. Infection, expander rupture or leakage, and disappointing outcomes are only a few examples of complications. Following post-operative care instructions to the letter and visiting the surgeon frequently are both crucial.

What to Expect Post-Procedure

Depending on the location being treated and the person's healing process, there might be a wide range in the time required for tissue expansion. However, a second treatment is carried out to remove the expander and finish the reconstruction after the desired amount of new skin has been produced.

Cost Factors

Tissue expanders are frequently utilized for reconstructive treatments, thus insurance may pay all or part of the price. However, this can differ significantly based on the insurance company and the particular circumstances.

Procedures using tissue expanders are essential weapons in the reconstructive plastic surgeon's toolbox because they enable more adaptable and successful results. A board-certified plastic surgeon's advice is essential before beginning any potential trip into the world of tissue expansion because everyone's needs and dangers are unique.

CHAPTER FOUR

4. Cosmetic Plastic Surgery for Men

Contrary to popular opinion, anyone can get plastic surgery. The many cosmetic surgeries that are available can help men as well, improving their appearance and raising their self-esteem. Men's aesthetic plastic surgery will be covered in detail in this chapter, including gynecomastia surgery, pectoral implants, jawline augmentation, abdominal etching, and hair transplants. We'll look at the reasons men choose to get plastic surgery, the difficulties they could encounter while recovering, and the effects these surgeries may have on their lives. This chapter will offer helpful insights and advice to assist you in making decisions, whether you're a male thinking about plastic surgery or are just curious about the possibilities.

Hair Transplant

In terms of looks, particularly for men, hair is crucial in determining self-esteem and confidence. The use of hair transplant procedures as the standard treatment for male-pattern baldness and other types of hair loss has been on the rise. It's an investment in your self-image; it's not just a surface alteration.

Understanding Hair Transplants

Hair follicles are transplanted onto bald or thinning areas during a hair transplant process from a donor site, which is typically the back or sides of your head. The procedure distributes the follicles in a way that replicates how hair grows naturally, aiming for a natural-looking outcome.

Is It Right For You?

A hair transplant may be appealing if you're struggling with thinning hair or receding hairlines. To serve as donor sites, however, good candidates often need robust hair growth on the sides and back of the head. Other elements that may affect the choice include age, the severity of hair loss, and expectations.

Techniques and Procedures

The two basic procedures are Follicular Unit Extraction (FUE) and Follicular Unit Transplantation (FUT). FUE harvests individual hair follicles, whereas FUT requires removing a strip of skin with hair follicles from the donor site. Both have advantages and disadvantages that you should properly consider with your surgeon (*Vogel et al., 2013*).

Financial Implications

Due to the aesthetic aspect of hair transplants, insurance typically does not cover them. The price varies according on the quantity of grafts required, the technique selected, and the surgeon's level of experience. It's critical to balance these aspects against the procedure's promised emotional and psychological advantages.

Risks and Side Effects

Swelling, pain, and momentary numbness are examples of typical adverse effects. Rare but probable are more severe consequences like infection or unnatural-looking hair growth. These dangers can be reduced with careful planning and an expert surgeon.

Long-Term Results

The durability of a hair transplant is one of its alluring qualities. The hair that has been transplanted typically grows for the rest of one's life once it starts. However, more treatments might be necessary, particularly if age-related natural hair loss persists.

Emotional Uplift

For many guys, growing out their hair restores more than just their youthful appearance. It improves their mental stability and self-esteem, which has a positive effect on a variety of daily activities, such as networking and career progress.

Post-Op Care

Post-operative care is simple yet essential. Antibiotics will probably be provided to you in order to prevent infection, and you might have to take a few weeks off from intense activity. To guarantee that the transplant is successful, proper scalp care and follow-up visits are necessary.

For males experiencing hair loss, a hair transplant offers a workable, long-term answer. This surgical journey can have a profound impact on your outlook on life, but it demands thoughtful consideration of your options and a dedication to post-operative care.

Abdominal Etching

Despite spending hours in the gym, getting sculpted abs remains a distant dream for many men. If you fit this description, abdominal etching might be the solution you've been looking for. It's more than just surgery; it's an artistic technique that improves the muscular tissue already present to produce more clearly defined abdominal muscles.

The Basics of Abdominal Etching

A type of liposuction called abdominal etching aims to enhance the look of muscular definition. To get a more chiseled appearance, the operation includes surgically eliminating fat from the areas surrounding the natural outlines of the muscles. Instead of building muscles, it reveals and enhances what already exists.

Who's the Ideal Candidate?

The people who are most suitable for this surgery are already in decent physical shape but have obstinate fat pockets that cover their abdominal muscles. This is not a weight-loss method like conventional liposuction. Instead, it's a technique for improving for those who are close to their optimal weight.

The How-to: Surgical Procedure

A local or general anesthetic is typically used for abdominal etching, which is typically done as an outpatient surgery. The abdomen's natural creases or the belly button are the sites of the surgeon's brief incisions. The extra fat is then removed from the area around your ab muscles using a cannula (*Sistemas e Publicações & Viaro, 2019*).

Financial Commitment

The cost of abdominal etching can vary depending on where you live and how complicated the procedure is. Insurance typically doesn't cover this operation because it is regarded as cosmetic. It's crucial to take into account not only the cost of the surgery but also any additional costs like anesthesia and post-operative care.

Potential Risks

Bruising, swelling, and transient numbness are typical concerns connected with this operation. Infection, scarring, and asymmetries are concerns that are more serious but less frequent. So it's crucial to pick a qualified and experienced surgeon.

After the Cut: Recovery and Results

Depending on how quickly each person heals and the complexity of the procedure, recovery time might range from a few days to several weeks. Typically, wearing compression clothing is advised to aid in the healing process. Despite being long-lasting, the results can be impacted by major weight changes. So, keeping the effects alive requires maintaining a steady weight and leading a healthy lifestyle.

Lifestyle Impact

The abdominal etching procedure has significant psychological advantages. Following the surgery, a significant confidence boost is felt by many guys. This improved self-esteem frequently spills over into other facets of life, such as social interactions and career chances.

A particular method of liposuction called abdominal etching provides a quick route to a torso with more definition. It has its own set of issues, from eligibility to recuperation, as with any surgical operation. The ultimate goal? A well-defined midsection that improves both your physical appearance and general quality of life.

Jawline Enhancement

Jawline augmentation may be worth looking into if you've ever thought your jawline lacks definition or could use some sharpening. It's a cosmetic surgery designed to reshape the lower face, giving the jawline and chin area definition and structure.

The Essence of Jawline Enhancement

The process may or may not involve surgery. Injectable fillers may be used as a non-surgical alternative to surgical procedures that frequently include implants or bone contouring techniques. Whatever method you use, the objective is to balance your facial characteristics and accentuate your jawline.

Candidate Credentials

Those who desire to achieve a more youthful appearance or boost their side profile become excellent candidates for jawline enlargement. However, realistic expectations are required, and general health is important. For a thorough facial study prior to moving forward, speak with your surgeon.

Procedural Steps

A biocompatible implant is frequently placed as part of a surgical improvement to give the jawline a more definite form. Injectable fillers, such as hyaluronic acid, can provide a less permanent but less intrusive alternative to surgery. Your decision will be influenced by your surgical readiness, financial situation, and cosmetic aspirations (*Harris & Raggio, 2022*).

Fiscal Aspects

The improvement of the jawline is typically not covered by insurance, as is frequently the case with elective cosmetic treatments. Depending on the approach and practitioner, prices can vary greatly. Make sure you account for both the upfront costs as well as any additional treatments or remedial procedures.

Consider the Risks

Despite being largely safe, potential dangers can include infections, asymmetry, and unhappiness with the appearance of the results. Additional issues in the case of surgery could be anesthetic risks and scars. So selecting a qualified surgeon is essential to reducing these dangers.

Journey of Recovery

Recovery from surgical procedures can take many weeks and be accompanied by bruising, swelling, and discomfort. Recovery from non-surgical procedures is typically rapid, with just mild side effects including slight swelling or bruising. For the best outcomes in both situations, full following to the post-procedure instructions is essential.

Impact on Self-Image

Undoubtedly, the process frequently results in a rise in confidence. Positive effects on both personal and professional interactions can be seen when you have a more defined jawline, which can change not only how you see yourself but also how others see you.

Procedures to improve the jawline provide a focused method for improving face appearance. These procedures can provide a long-lasting fix for the lower face's lack of definition or structure by enhancing or reshaping the jaw. Understanding the range of alternatives, potential dangers, and recovery expectations will help you make an informed choice if you're thinking about getting a more defined jawline.

Pectoral Implants

Although exercises and gym visits may provide a path to a sculpted chest, they aren't always sufficient. Pectoral implants offer a fascinating alternative for individuals looking for results that are more certain. This surgical procedure, which aims to increase the size and improve the contour of the chest muscles, is becoming more and more popular among men who want to look more chiseled.

What are Pectoral Implants?

These biocompatible silicone implants were created specifically to enlarge the male chest. These silicone implants, which are solid unlike the breast implants used by women, give the appearance of being firmer and more muscular. During a surgical operation, they are positioned beneath the pre-existing pectoral muscles.

Who Stands to Benefit?

Men who, despite regular exercise, are unable to acquire the size or fullness of their ideal chest might consider pectoral implants. This technique provides a solution to a more balanced, aesthetically acceptable upper torso for people who have congenital or acquired chest wall abnormalities.

The Process

The procedure is typically carried out while the patient is asleep. The surgeon makes an incision in the armpit through which he or she makes a pocket under the pectoral muscle. After that, the implant is placed for best aesthetic results. The wounds are stitched up, typically with dissolvable sutures (*Benito-Ruiz et al., 2007*).

Budgetary Matters

The cost of pectoral implants is comparable to that of other cosmetic treatments. Anesthesia costs, hospital fees, and surgeon fees are a few examples of the variables that can affect the price. Keep in mind that insurance rarely pays for cosmetic surgery, so you should have a budget in place.

Risk Factors

Complications can happen even if they are comparatively uncommon. Infection, implant displacement, and capsular contracture (tissue hardening around the implant) are all possible complications. Before undergoing any procedure, always go over the risks and your concerns with your surgeon.

What to Expect After Surgery

Swelling, bruising, and soreness during the early stages of recovery are typical; these symptoms can be controlled with medicine. For several weeks, physical activity will be limited, especially for the upper body.

Long-term Results and Self-Image

Your chest will remain more muscular for a long time because the implants are made to last. To maintain the general appearance of your chest, your lifestyle decisions, such as nutrition and exercise, will be important.

For guys who want a larger, more muscular chest, pectoral implants are an alternative. These implants can be placed through a simple operation and provide long-lasting benefits, letting you flaunt your self-assurance even when the weather is cool. Despite the financial investment and surgical risks required to achieve this improved physique, for many people the increase in self-esteem and bodily pleasure makes the trip worthwhile.

Liposuction

Despite consistent exercise and strict eating habits, body fat can be a tenacious foe that sticks to certain locations. Men can benefit from liposuction as a surgical option that can remove fat from specific places and shape body parts that may not respond to conventional weight loss techniques.

What is Liposuction?

A cosmetic surgery called liposuction involves sucking off fat deposits from certain body parts. The neck, chest, love handles, and belly are typical target areas for guys. The technique can be used to treat benign fatty tumors called lipomas or for solely cosmetic reasons.

Who's an Ideal Candidate?

The greatest candidates are typically males who are close to their desired weight but unable to lose fat from particular problem regions. It's also critical to have reasonable expectations and recognize that liposuction is a body-contouring operation rather than a weight-loss method.

How It's Done

The surgeon will perform minor incisions in the desired location after providing anaesthetic. Then, to break apart and suck out fat, a thin tube known as a cannula is inserted. Depending on the location and volume of fat being removed, the approach may change, and tools like lasers or ultrasound may be employed to speed up the procedure (*Saad et al., 2020*).

Price Tag and Financing

Since liposuction is a cosmetic procedure that is electively chosen, health insurance frequently does not pay for it. The price may change depending on the experience and reputation of the operating surgeon, the facility's proximity to the patient, and the degree of difficulty of the operation. Make sure you plan your finances appropriately, and if necessary, look into financing possibilities.

Risks and Recovery

As with any operation, there are inherent dangers, such as the possibility of infection, hemorrhage, or a negative anesthetic reaction. For the first few weeks after surgery, it is recommended that patients rest and wear a compression garment. Be prepared for some swelling and bruising, which should progressively go away.

Long-lasting Impact

The treated areas undergo a lasting alteration since the eliminated fat cells cannot regrow. However, it's crucial to keep your weight steady after surgery because big swings can affect the outcomes.

Mind the Mirror

This process has the power to transform one's confidence and self-perception. Even though it might not be able to completely replace the requirement for a healthy lifestyle, it can be a huge help in your quest for a more chiseled body.

Male liposuction offers a successful, albeit surgically invasive, method of eliminating stubborn fat and improving physical features. Although it has its share of costs and hazards, the assurance and satisfaction it may provide are frequently thought to be well worth the expenditure.

Penis Enhancement

It is inevitable that the subject of penis augmentation comes up while talking about plastic surgery for guys. Given that it touches on delicate issues of male identity and body image, this surgery may spark both interest and controversy. Here, we take a closer look at what penile augmentation surgery includes and who is a good candidate for it.

What Is Penis Enhancement?

Penis enhancement, commonly referred to as penile enlargement surgery, tries to lengthen or widen the penis, or both. The procedure may involve a variety of procedures, such as removing ligaments or grafting fat cells from different body regions. Surgical treatments for disorders like Peyronie's disease and hypospadias are not to be confused with this.

The Right Candidate: Who Stands to Benefit?

Many men who contemplate this procedure worry that their penis size may negatively impact their sexual confidence or their ability to find a romantic partner. It's important to remember that many guys overestimate what is 'normal' and may not require surgery. The first step in determining eligibility is a thorough consultation with a licensed surgeon.

Techniques Explored

There are various ways to improve the penis, each having benefits and cons. By transferring fat from one area of the body to the penis, autologous fat grafting increases penile girth. Another method, known as ligamentolysis, releases the suspensory ligament to lengthen the penis, albeit this might occasionally change the angle at which it erections (*Littara et al., 2019*).

Financial Aspects

This surgery is usually not covered by insurance because it is elective. Expenses can differ substantially based on variables like the nature of the procedure, the skill level of the surgeon, and the patient's location. It's important to talk openly about the charges and any prospective supplemental expenses like further treatments or changes.

Risks and Aftercare

Penis augmentation carries dangers like infection, scars, and unhappiness with outcomes, just like any surgical procedure. You could be required to follow cleanliness and pharmaceutical instructions during the postoperative period, as well as refrain from sexual activity for a predetermined amount of time.

Longevity of Results

Depending on the method employed and personal circumstances like weight growth or aging, the benefits may not last as long as desired. While some techniques provide longer-lasting results, none can provide eternal youth or unending dimensions.

Societal and Psychological Impacts

Even though the operation can result in a noticeable size difference, the psychological effects shouldn't be understated. As this is a treatment that tries to improve not only anatomy, but also self-perception and confidence, it is crucial that all parties involved have realistic expectations and are well aware of the hazards involved.

The decision to have penis augmentation surgery is complex and subtle, needing thorough research. Its effects extend beyond purely bodily modifications and touch upon society standards and psychological wellbeing. As a result, it must always be tackled carefully, with professional advice, and with considerable investigation.

Gynecomastia Surgery

Gynecomastia is a disorder that sparks a lot of debate but is seldom discussed in public. Gynecomastia, a condition that causes male breast tissue to grow, can cause significant emotional discomfort and self-consciousness.

Defining Gynecomastia Surgery

Reduction mammoplasty, another name for gynecomastia surgery, is a treatment used to shrink oversized male breasts. In some situations, extra skin, fat, and breast tissue are also removed during the procedure. The removal of tissue could be combined with liposuction.

Why Opt for Surgery?

Gynecomastia can sometimes go away on its own or with medicine, but persistent cases frequently prompt people to think about having surgery. When alternative treatments have failed and the problem has stabilized—that is, there hasn't been any change in breast size for at least a year—surgery becomes a possible choice.

Are You a Candidate?

Gynecomastia surgery candidates often have good general health, stable weight, and reasonable expectations. To get the best outcomes, skin elasticity must be in good shape because low elasticity could impair the skin's capacity to retract after surgery.

Types of Procedures

Different surgical techniques may be utilized, depending on the severity of gynecomastia. In situations where excessive fatty tissue is the main issue, liposuction alone may be sufficient. However, excision procedures are typically needed for larger glandular tissue (*Holzmer et al., 2020*).

What to Expect Post-Surgery

In order to reduce swelling and support the new chest contour following surgery, patients can often anticipate wearing a compression garment. Although common, pain can be controlled with prescribed medicine. Most people can go back to work in a week and begin physically demanding activities in approximately a month.

Cost Considerations

Gynecomastia surgery can come at a hefty financial cost. The cost will vary depending on the procedure's specifics, the surgeon's experience, and the patient's location. Insurance might not pay the fees because it's frequently regarded as cosmetic.

Risks and Complications

Infection, scarring, and an uneven chest shape are typical complications. The nipple may also experience alterations in its sensory function. Always explore these potential hazards in detail at a full consultation with your physician.

Lasting Impact

Gynecomastia surgery frequently has benefits that reach beyond the body. Following surgery, a lot of guys say they feel better about themselves and have a more positive self-image. Preserving the outcomes of surgery requires a commitment to a healthy lifestyle, as factors such as weight increase and hormonal changes might lead to a return of the condition.

When addressing gynecomastia, surgery offers a long-term remedy for people who discover that the issue significantly lowers their quality of life. As with any surgery, making well-informed decisions and following expert advice are crucial.

Botox and Fillers

Non-surgical cosmetic procedures like Botox and dermal fillers haven't merely been used by women in recent years to seem younger. Men are increasingly exploring this area as well, drawn by the prospect of small alterations with little downtime. Let's analyze the subtleties of this world of injectables for guys.

Understanding Botox and Fillers

In order to cure wrinkles brought on by muscular activity, such as frown lines and crow's feet, a kind of botulinum toxin known as "Botox" is typically employed. The goal of fillers, on the other hand, is to restore volume to regions where it has been lost over time. Fillers are gel-like substances like hyaluronic acid or collagen. Muscles are "frozen" by botox while skin is "plumped up" by fillers—two separate but occasionally complementing goals.

Why the Growing Interest Among Men?

Due to the societal stigmas being lessened and a greater understanding of the need of preserving looks, more men are choosing non-invasive cosmetic operations. Additionally, compared to surgical procedures, its effects are simpler to reverse and the operation is typically short and straightforward (*Lem et al., 2023*).

Who's a Candidate?

You're probably an excellent candidate if you have fine lines that look more like trenches or facial volume loss that gives you a worn-out, drawn-out appearance. To find out what's appropriate for your unique circumstances, it's imperative to speak with a qualified professional.

Different Products, Different Goals

Dynamic wrinkles, or those caused by muscular activity, are frequently treated with Botox. Static wrinkles—which are noticeable even when your face is relaxed—are the kind of wrinkles that fillers are more frequently utilized for. Other uses for them include enhancing the lips, enhancing the cheeks, and even contouring the jawline.

What About Risks?

Botox and fillers are generally safe when used by a trained professional, but they do have some dangers, such as the possibility of bruising, infection, or an allergic response. There is a slight possibility of eyelid or brow drooping after receiving Botox. Sometimes fillers can cause lumpiness or asymmetry. Remember to share any worries you have with your healthcare professional.

After the Procedure

These therapies involve very little downtime. Despite some little swelling or redness, you can usually resume your day practically soon. When compared to fillers, which can last anywhere from six months to two years, Botox results are visible within a week and can last up to four months.

Let's Talk Budget

Botox and fillers aren't exactly inexpensive, though they are less expensive than the majority of surgical treatments. Depending on the region and provider's skill, prices can vary greatly. These procedures are rarely covered by insurance since they are considered cosmetic.

Botox and fillers give men a range of alternatives for aesthetic refinement, whether it's to smooth out a wrinkle here or add some volume there. It's a less intimidating way to go into the world of aesthetic improvements, and individuals who aren't quite ready for more invasive operations may find it particularly alluring. Just keep in mind that meticulous planning and expert execution are the keys to success.

Laser Treatments

Men are increasingly turning to laser procedures, which are gradually becoming as the preferred choice for those seeking minimally invasive procedures with minimal side effects. These cutting-edge techniques promise skin condition improvement and even regeneration. Let's explore the diverse world of laser treatments for men, from getting rid of unwanted hair to treating acne scars.

The What and How of Laser Treatments

Lasers are concentrated light beams that pierce the skin without harming the top layer. To target particular skin disorders, many types of lasers—including fractional, IPL, and Q-Switched—operate at various wavelengths and serve various purposes. Some lasers work well to remove pigmentation, while others are better suited to treating wrinkles or slack skin.

Why Men Are Opting for Lasers

Convenience in a nutshell. Most laser treatment sessions last around an hour, making them quick procedures. You can nearly leave the clinic and continue with your day because there is little to no downtime. Furthermore, they provide a degree of precision that conventional treatments frequently cannot match.

Suitability: Is It for You?

What you're seeking to accomplish will largely determine if you're a candidate for laser treatments. Want to get rid of sun damage or age spots? A laser can be used for that. Looking to reduce acne scars or fine lines? It can be handled by lasers. To fully grasp the variety of alternatives and how they relate to your unique circumstances, always begin with a consultation.

Safety Concerns and Risks

There are hazards associated with laser treatments, just like with other medical procedure. These can be as innocuous as some redness and swelling, or as dangerous as an infection, burn, or even a change in skin color. These hazards will be greatly reduced by selecting a licensed specialist for the treatment (*Lem et al., 2023*).

The Price Tag: What to Expect

The cost of laser treatments is high. You should be prepared to spend anywhere between a few hundred and several thousand dollars, depending on the type of laser being used and the area being treated. Also keep in mind that certain treatments need numerous sessions to produce the best results; plan your budget appropriately.

Post-Procedure Life

For one or two days following the procedure, the treated area may experience symptoms like a mild sunburn. You'll probably be told to refrain from strenuous activity and prolonged sun exposure. For long-lasting outcomes, further sessions can be required, and a maintenance schedule might be suggested for particular problems.

Men's laser treatments are gaining popularity as a safe substitute for more intrusive procedures since they offer a variety of alternatives for treating different skin problems. Despite the initial cost, many people find it to be an appealing option due to its simplicity and effectiveness. But like with any medical choice, it's essential to speak with a licensed expert, not only for safety but also to make sure you're spending money on a course of action that's actually in line with your objectives.

CHAPTER FIVE

5. Reconstructive Plastic Surgery for Men

Reconstructive plastic surgery can improve function and appearance following injury, illness, or congenital deformities in both men and women. The special difficulties that men who have reconstructive plastic surgery must overcome will be the main topic of this chapter. These difficulties include male breast reduction, scar revision, burn reconstruction, earlobe repair, hand surgery, and cleft lip repair. We'll look at the many methods applied in these surgeries, the healing procedures, and the psychological effects they may have on males. We hope to increase awareness of these lesser-known procedures and inspire men to get the support they require to go above their physical obstacles and enhance their overall quality of life by showcasing them.

Male Breast Reduction

Male breast reduction has a unique place in the complex world of plastic surgery. Despite the fact that most people only think of males when they talk about breast surgery, there has been a rise in the number of guys seeking treatment for gynecomastia. Loss of self-esteem can result from this illness, which can also have an impact on one's mental health in addition to their physical look.

What Male Breast Reduction Is All About

Male breast reduction, often known as gynecomastia surgery, is a technique designed to treat males with oversized or excessively developed breasts. The procedure often entails liposuction to remove extra fat, and excision methods may also be necessary to remove glandular tissue or extra skin. The operation rebuilds not only the shape but also the confidence by restoring a flatter, firmer, and more manly chest contour (*Plastic Surgery for Gynecomastia: Practice Essentials, History of the Procedure, Problem, 2023*).

What Triggers the Need?

Gynecomastia can develop for a variety of reasons, from hormonal abnormalities to drug adverse effects. It is also recognized that aging, weight growth, and particular medical disorders are to blame. Gynecomastia can physically hurt, causing breast tenderness in addition to just being unsightly. It often becomes essential for both physical and mental wellbeing to address these issues.

Getting Through the Pre-Surgery Maze

It is common practice to do a thorough medical evaluation before beginning the surgical process. In order to rule out any cancers, this may involve blood tests, mammograms, and occasionally even biopsies. The key to a successful outcome is open communication between you and your surgeon regarding your goals, potential risks, and advantages.

Operational Tactics: The Procedure

Typically, the operation is an outpatient procedure that lasts about 90 minutes. The surgeon does liposuction to remove extra fat after giving anesthetic. Depending on each individual case, glandular tissue or excess skin may also need to be removed. To reduce obvious scars, the incisions are subsequently sewn up and frequently blended into the natural curves of the chest.

Recovery: The Road to Your New Self

You can anticipate some stiffness, swelling, and bruising following the procedure, but these side effects often go away in a few weeks. It is frequently advised to wear a compression garment to promote the healing process and aid decrease edema. For at least three to four weeks following surgery, physical activity should be avoided, particularly those involving upper body movements. You will be scheduled for routine checkups and perhaps some imaging tests to track your healing and outcomes.

Cost and Insurance Coverage

It costs money to have a male breast reduction. Depending on the surgeon's skill, the complexity of the treatment, and the patient's location, prices might range from $3,000 to $8,000. The price of the procedure might be covered by health insurance if it is medically essential, however the majority of cosmetic instances are not covered by insurance.

Long-Term Outcomes: Embrace the Change

Surgery results are typically long-lasting when realistic expectations are maintained and postoperative instructions are followed. The results can be substantially prolonged by maintaining a steady weight and leading a healthy lifestyle. To avoid a recurrence of gynecomastia, it's important to be aware of the possibility of any considerable weight gain, hormone imbalances, or drug use.

The transformational nature of male breast reduction goes beyond just aesthetics. This is a chance to put money into yourself and get your life back in shape, both physically and mentally. But in order to make sure you're making a wise and advantageous choice, it's essential to approach it with the proper attitude and under competent direction.

Scar Revision

While scars may serve as physical reminders of a variety of experiences or events in life, not everyone views them as beautiful artifacts. For some people, a scar may serve as an ongoing reminder of a traumatic event or may just be an unsightly mark that affects one's self-image. The solution is scar revision surgery, a specialist operation designed to reduce the scar's visual impact and better integrate it with the skin and texture around it.

The Anatomy of Scar Revision

Scar revision aims to reduce the scar's visibility rather than completely remove it. This surgical procedure entails removing the scar tissue and carefully stitching the new wound, frequently using cutting-edge methods to move the scar to a less noticeable location or change its shape. The scar can be concealed using a number of techniques, including Z-plasty, W-plasty, and geometric broken line closure.

Why Consider Scar Revision?

Considerations for scar remodeling might range from worries about appearance to problems with functionality. Some scars, particularly those that overlap joints or are on the face, might limit motion and even cause pain. A person's ability to negotiate social circumstances and their view of themselves can be negatively impacted by emotional scars that carry the burden of self-consciousness.

Preparing for the Procedure

An extensive consultation with a licensed plastic surgeon is required prior to beginning scar correction. They will assess the scar, go through your expectations, and describe the surgical choices that are most appropriate in your situation. Certain drugs or smoking may be prohibited prior to surgery as these can have an impact on the healing process.

The Nuts and Bolts: Procedure Insights

Depending on the form and location of the scar, the procedure's length varies, but it's typically an outpatient experience. Depending on the scope of the operation, either local or general anesthetic will be given. The surgeon may use additional procedures like dermabrasion or laser therapy after the excision and suturing to further improve the texture and look of the scar (*Garg et al., 2014*).

Journey to Recovery

After the procedure, the operated area should experience some edema, soreness, and redness. Antibiotics and painkillers are frequently administered to treat discomfort and avoid infection. For best results, it is essential to adhere to your surgeon's aftercare recommendations, including any suggested topical treatments.

Financial Considerations

Scar revision costs can vary significantly, depending on the complexity of the treatment, the facility fees, and the surgeon's experience. Purely cosmetic scar revision is often not covered by insurance, but functional limitations brought on by scarring may be covered.

Sustaining the Results

The full results take time to develop as the new scar ages and fades, while there are some instant benefits that can be seen. Maintaining a strict aftercare routine that includes moisturizing and sun protection can improve and extend the results.

Scar revision gives you a second opportunity and a chance to slightly alter your story. By being proactive and being guided by professional knowledge, you are changing more than simply a patch of skin; one mark at a time, you are changing how you show yourself to the world.

Burn Reconstruction

An emotional ordeal like a burn injury, which leaves permanent physical and emotional scars, is more than just a medical ailment. The chance for victims to restore their lives and looks is provided by breakthroughs in reconstructive surgery, which is a ray of hope. The field of burn reconstruction combines medical expertise with human resiliency to make the seemingly impossible appear practically achievable.

The Anatomy of Burn Reconstruction

Each patient undergoing burn reconstruction surgery will have a procedure that is specific to their condition and designed to restore as much of their normal appearance as possible. The secret is in repairing not only the surface layers, but all the way down to the underlying structures. Skin grafts, tissue expansion, reconstructive flaps, and even microsurgery may be used in more severe situations.

Why Burn Reconstruction?

Burn scars are not only unsightly, but they can also be functionally disabling, causing limited mobility and even organ dysfunction in extreme situations. Reconstruction is motivated by more than simply improving one's appearance; it's also driven by improving one's general well-being and ability to carry out daily tasks.

Pre-Operative Evaluation

The first stage is a thorough consultation with the plastic surgeon to discuss the patient's medical and mental preparations for the procedure. The surgeon will describe the available surgical choices, any possible dangers, and the anticipated results. The initial burn wounds' progress toward healing and the patient's general state of health determine when the surgery will take place.

Behind the Scalpel: The Procedures

One of the most popular methods is skin grafting, which involves moving healthy skin from another region of the body to the burned area. Another common technique is tissue expansion, which enables the body to 'create' additional skin that is then utilized to replace the burned or scarred skin. Free flaps, which involve transferring skin from another area of the body along with its blood supply, may be required in more complicated circumstances (*Klein et al., 2007*).

The Recovery Voyage

Depending on how extensive the surgery was, the early aftermath of burn reconstruction could need a hospital stay. In the recovery period, it's crucial to control pain, take care of the wounds, and guard against infection. The recovery process frequently includes physical and occupational therapy, especially when the burn affects mobility.

A Financial Palette

Burn rebuilding is a multiphase process that can be expensive. If the surgery is deemed medically necessary rather than merely aesthetic, insurance companies may cover part or all aspects of the care.

Longevity of Results

Burn reconstruction is frequently a drawn-out process needing numerous surgeries and long-term aftercare, even though the main objective is to enhance both aesthetics and functionality. Results are often long-lasting but can be affected by a variety of things, including lifestyle decisions, aging, and general health.

Reconstructing someone's life and sense of self after a severe burn takes more than simply a medical treatment. It serves as evidence for the power of medical advancements combined with unwavering human determination to systematically reshape society.

Earlobe Repair

The impact of earlobe repair on one's sense of self-worth and one's sense of aesthetic appeal is undeniable, but it may not get as much press as other, more complex surgeries. This treatment is the hidden hero of tiny but significant cosmetic alterations, whether it be caused by intentional earlobe stretching or injury from a pulled earring.

The Why of Earlobe Repair

The majority of people who need their earlobes repaired have either intentionally or accidentally torn them from wearing earrings. Over time, elongation may also be caused by ordinary wear and strain. In addition to repairing the damage, a simple fix here enables the ears to be re-pierced, restoring the ability to wear those eye-catching accessories.

The Anatomy of the Repair

Each earlobe repair is personalized to fit the patient's particular circumstances; this is not an assembly line. An earlobe's natural contours are often preserved by delicate stitching after the surgeon carefully eliminates any strained or torn tissue. The use of local anesthetic guarantees an almost pain-free experience.

Procedure Nuances

The surgical approach depends on the type of tear. Sometimes only a few small stitches are needed to mend incomplete rips. Skin around full tears or more severe stretching would need to be removed, then the earlobe's form would need to be aligned with sutures. In cases of severe stretching, the restoration may be more difficult and require the reshaping of both the lobe and surrounding parts of the ear (*Sadaka & Bakr Hantash, 2022*).

Road to Recovery

Earlobe repair requires quite minimal post-operative care. Most patients are given a prescription for a light painkiller and antibiotics to prevent infection, and they are free to leave the hospital the same day. Although swelling and redness following surgery are common, they usually go away within a few days. After a week or two, sutures are typically removed, and a new piercing can be contemplated.

Financial Footnote

In general, earlobe repair is less expensive than other cosmetic procedures. It's crucial to determine whether your insurance company views the operation as medically necessary because it would affect coverage. If not, a lot of clinics provide flexible payment options.

The Legacy of Earlobe Repair

Even though you may think, "It's just an earlobe," the aesthetic and practical advantages are real. Following the operation, earrings can once again be worn because the ear's natural symmetry is restored. Despite being a minor body component, the earlobe's appearance has a considerable impact on face harmony and self-esteem.

Earlobe repair serves as a model for how small modifications may have a big impact because of its exquisite simplicity. It may not be an operation that changes your life, but for many people, it's an essential first step towards feeling normal and satisfied with your appearance.

Hand Surgery

A hand is more than just a physical component of your body; it is a tool that engages with the outside world and has a variety of effects on how you live your life. Its significance cannot be emphasized, from holding a pen to shaking hands. The recovery of functional autonomy and personal freedom through hand surgery is therefore more than just a physical restoration.

Why Opt for Hand Surgery?

Conditions present at birth, trauma, and degenerative diseases like arthritis are only some of the reasons to seek hand surgery. Hand surgery can be life-changing, whether it's regaining movement after an accident or treating a longstanding abnormality. Candidate's quality of life is frequently hampered by poor functionality, persistent pain, or aesthetic problems.

The Types and Techniques

The field of hand surgery is wide and includes a variety of specialist treatments. Only a few examples include fracture fixations, joint replacements, tendon repairs, and carpal tunnel release. The surgical strategy will be determined by the particular ailment, necessitating a personalized treatment plan. Techniques could range from open surgeries with larger incisions to minimally invasive arthroscopic procedures (*Tuaño et al., 2023*).

Navigating the Surgical Maze

In many cases, a team of specialists, including the surgeon, radiologist, physical therapist, and rheumatologist, is required to achieve the best possible outcome. Diagnostic imaging can identify the problem, and preoperative discussions will go over the risks, advantages, and expected rates of recovery. Personalization is essential because no two hand operations are alike.

Post-Op Pathway

The hand may need to be immobilized during the post-operative period, and analgesics and antibiotics may be prescribed to treat any lingering discomfort and infections. For optimum recovery, rehabilitation must start as soon as possible. Within days of surgery, physical therapy is typically started with the goal of restoring strength and function. It is advised to gradually resume everyday activities while being closely monitored by routine follow-up sessions.

The Economics of Hand Surgery

Depending on the complexity, location, and insurance coverage, hand surgery can be very expensive. Examining your policy carefully is essential to establish whether the procedure is considered medically necessary, which could affect insurance coverage. For patients to afford the operation, several surgical facilities provide payment options.

The Lingering Impact

Although hand surgery may seem intimidating, the long-term benefits are priceless. It is impossible to overstate the emotional and psychological boost, which goes beyond the physical alleviation. Well-being and self-esteem are impacted by achieving range of motion that was previously unattainable or going back to work after a protracted hiatus.

In the end, hand surgery is more than simply a medical procedure; it's a commitment to raising your standard of living. This serves to further emphasize the important truth that the path to self-fulfillment frequently starts with us literally taking responsibility for our own health.

Cleft Lip Repair in Men

Let's take a time to reflect on what a grin represents; it is more than simply an expression; it is a universal language that conveys happiness, self-assurance, and social connectivity. This straightforward action can come with a complex mix of practical and emotional concerns for males who were born with a cleft lip. The goal of cleft lip restoration for men is to redefine social interaction and self-esteem, not merely in terms of beauty.

The Groundwork: What Is Cleft Lip in Men?

A physical split in the top lip is a defining feature of the congenital disorder known as a cleft lip. It may happen on one side or both, and it might or might not affect the palate. Although typically rectified in childhood, adult males may need initial or revision surgery for a variety of factors, including reduced scarring and enhanced lip function.

Why Choose Repair?

For a variety of reasons, adult males may want to undergo cleft lip correction. The surgery can improve speech, feeding, and even respiratory efficiency in addition to cosmetic changes. Additionally, there may be a significant knock-on effect on psychological health, affecting everything from close relationships to professional accomplishments.

The Procedural Landscape

Adult cleft lip repair surgery can be more difficult than pediatric treatments, frequently requiring a multidisciplinary approach comprising psychologists, otolaryngologists, and oral surgeons. The anatomy and goals of each patient are taken into account while deciding which surgical technique, such as rotational advancement, straight line repair, or triangular flap, to use (*Adenwalla & Narayanan, 2009*).

Life After the Knife: Recovery and Beyond

Following surgery, the recuperation phase may require wound care, the administration of antibiotics, and restricted physical activity to avoid stressing the lip's healing process. As the surgical correction may change the structural dynamics of the mouth, patient-specific aftercare may entail speech therapy or orthodontic treatments.

Cost Considerations

The cost of treating an adult with a cleft lip might differ greatly. The difficulty of the surgery, the location, and the extent of post-operative care required are all factors. Certain insurance plans might provide only a portion of the cost of the surgery, particularly if it is judged medically required rather than merely aesthetic.

The Long Game: Reaping the Rewards

Although the full benefits take months or even years to materialize, the initial effects are sometimes noticeable within weeks. These are not limited to the mirror; they also reverberate in daily activities, social interactions, and even professional advancements. A cleft lip repair that goes well can have far-reaching effects on a person's quality of life, far beyond the immediate cosmetic benefits.

Men's cleft lip correction is more than just surgery; it's a total makeover that focuses on usefulness, aesthetics, and emotional balance. It involves rebuilding a broader, more self-assured you, not just fixing a broken part of you. After all, if one grin can convey so much, just think of what recovering yours could.

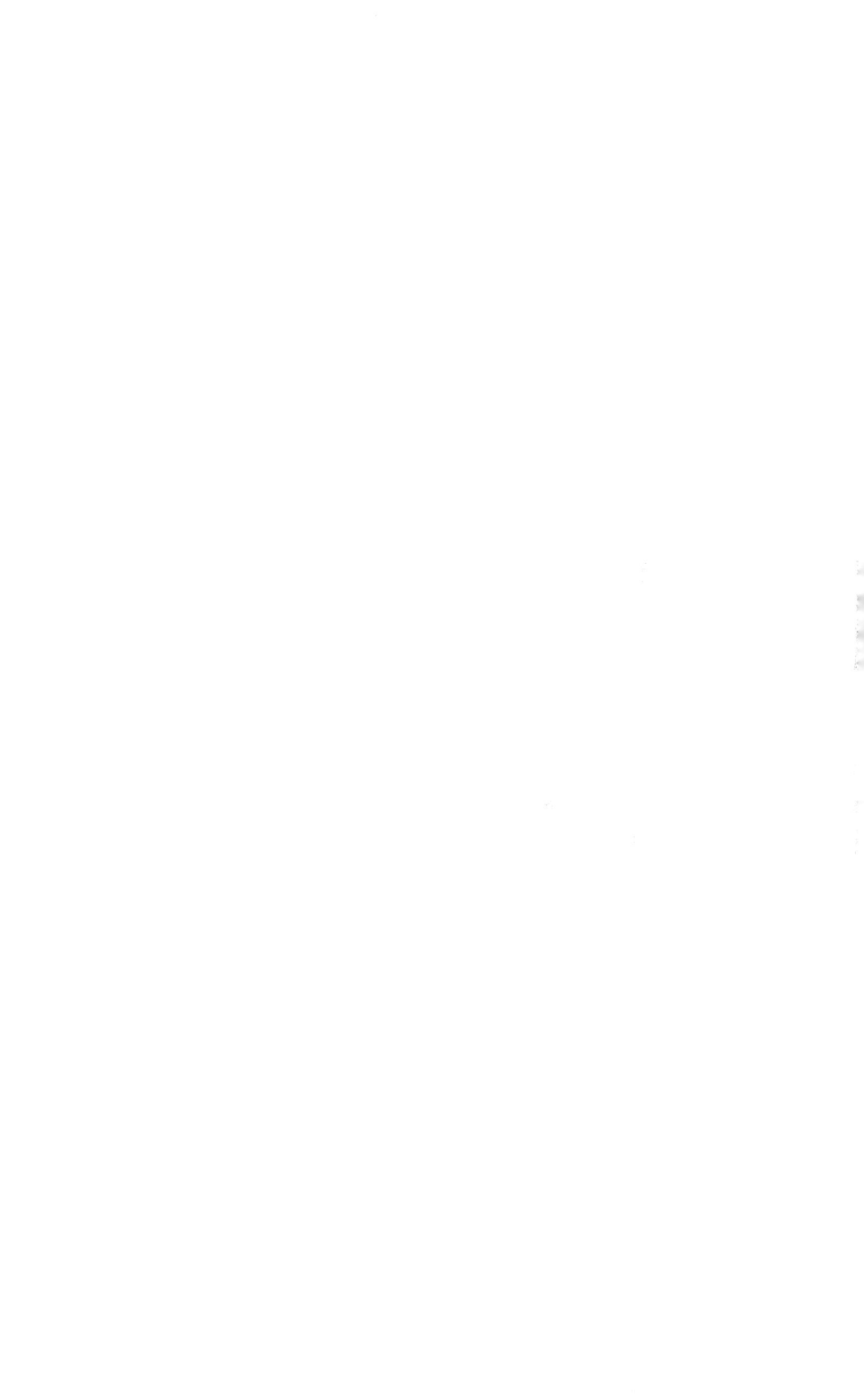

CHAPTER SIX

6. *Aesthetic Dermatology Treatments*

Our appearance and self-confidence may be impacted by the myriad changes that our skin goes through as we age. It's understandable to wish to turn back time and recover a young glow when you have ugly moles, age spots, fine lines, and wrinkles. While plastic surgery can produce impressive results, there are occasions when a less intrusive method is sufficient to produce the desired appearance.

Without requiring surgery, aesthetic dermatology procedures can improve the skin in a subtle but effective way. Non-invasive methods such as laser hair removal, cellulite treatment, RF microneedling, and mole removal are explored in this chapter. We'll go over the advantages, dangers, and healing times related to each therapy so you can decide on your skincare requirements with knowledge.

Mole Removal

From a medical standpoint, moles are essentially benign skin growths caused by a conglomeration of melanocytes, the pigment-producing cells. Their relevance goes beyond the purely clinical, though. In our daily lives, they frequently play a variety of roles, from identifiers ("Oh, you mean Sarah, with the mole on her cheek?") to Marilyn Monroe-style beauty markings. These seemingly harmless patches, however, might cause pain or self-consciousness for some people. Mole removal is an easy process that can have a major psychological influence on how you feel about your physical appearance.

The Nature of Moles: Harmless or Cause for Concern?

Not every mole is the same. They appear in a variety of shapes, sizes, and colors, and the majority of them never become health problems. However, some of them can bleed, itch, or—more seriously—develop into skin cancer. Mole removal provides a permanent treatment, whether it is required for medical or aesthetic reasons.

Why Mole Removal?

Medical professionals may advise mole removal if the mole exhibits signs of cancer or if it is causing physical discomfort. Remove a mole for cosmetic reasons if you think it unattractive or if its location (on your face or neck, for example) causes you to feel self-conscious. It boils down to a choice between your health and how you want to see yourself.

Your Options Unveiled: Types of Mole Removal Techniques

There are various methods to bid an unwanted mole farewell. While a surgical shave uses a knife to take off prominent moles, a surgical excision entails removing the mole plus a margin of the surrounding skin. Cryotherapy (freezing the mole) and laser mole removal are both options for people who are apprehensive about having surgery *(Bandral et al., 2018)*.

Anticipating the Journey: Pre-Procedure Consultation

A dermatologist will assess the mole before the surgery to choose the most effective removal technique. To exclude the risk of malignancy, a biopsy may be advised in specific circumstances. Your medical background, any prior skin issues, and what to anticipate following the surgery will also be covered.

The Recovery Narrative

Most of the time, recovery is simple and simply requires basic wound care. Depending on the technique employed, you might feel some little discomfort, scars, or discolouration, all of which typically go away over time. To reduce any hazards, it's essential to strictly adhere to your doctor's postoperative advice.

Pocket Impact: What Does Mole Removal Cost?

The cost of mole removal might vary depending on the method used, the size and location of the mole, and regional price variances. While aesthetic mole removals typically aren't, medical mole removals are frequently reimbursed by insurance.

The decision to remove moles is complex and affects both one's health and appearance. It goes beyond just cosmetic vanity. The process is often simple, with advantages that may be felt as well as seen, whether it is being done out of necessity for medical reasons or the desire for smoother skin. Imagine it as changing the story that is written on your skin, giving you control over how you are perceived by others. Making way for a new section of your tale rather than eliminating a significant portion of who you are.

Age Spot Removal

Age spots, sometimes referred to as sunspots or liver spots, are those unharmful, flat, brown blemishes that develop on the skin, frequently in locations that are exposed to the sun the most. Although they are primarily a sign of a life well lived—of countless summers and outdoor pursuits—they can occasionally feel like unwelcome guests, especially when they become exceptionally conspicuous or numerous. Age spot removal offers a cosmetic reset for those who feel that these spots conflict with their sense of self.

Age Spots

Age spots, a common consequence of aging and the sun's ultraviolet rays, typically make their first appearance in one's 40s or later. The choice to remove them can be motivated by aesthetic preferences or even the simple need for a change, even when they don't present any health risks.

Deciding on Age Spot Removal

Why take the risk? Some people find that these blemishes conflict with their personal look or act as an unwanted sign of age. Others could be concerned with getting a skin tone that is more even. Whatever the cause, the choice is entirely up to you. A dermatologist consultation can provide insightful information, but ultimately, the decision is up to the individual.

Techniques for Age Spot Removal

One of a number of procedures, each suited to particular requirements and skin types, may be recommended by your dermatologist. Melanin is the target of laser therapy, which also diffuses pigment clumps. In a chemical peel, an acid is applied to your skin, burning off the top layer to reveal new, healthy skin. The outermost layer of your skin is removed by a machine during microdermabrasion. Liquid nitrogen is used in cryotherapy, a less popular technique, to freeze the age spot (*Arora et al., 2012*).

The Prep Work

A doctor consultation is required before having any of these operations in order to go through your eligibility, the associated fees, and any possible adverse effects. You might have to stop taking some drugs or avoid getting too much sun as a result of some procedures.

Post-Treatment Care and Recovery

Depending on the approach taken, recovery may differ. While chemical peels may take up to a week to fully recover from, laser therapy may leave your skin red for a few hours. During the healing process, moisturizing and sunscreen are vital components of skincare.

Cost Factor

Depending on the procedure employed and the quantity of sessions needed, the cost can vary significantly. Age spot removal is typically seen as cosmetic and is not supported by health insurance. However, the price is frequently comparable to the psychological advantage of better self-esteem.

Removing age spots is less about "turning back the clock" and more about taking control of the scars left by your encounters with the world. What counts most is how the decision fits into your own, individual story, regardless of whether the need for removal is motivated by vanity or a desire for conformity. It has never been easier to have the freedom to sculpt this chapter of your life story thanks to the plethora of techniques at your disposal.

Chemical Peels

It's not always about keeping what you already have; sometimes, skincare involves pressing the reset button. Chemical peels can give your skin a serious restart by drastically enhancing its tone, texture, and overall look. How do chemical peels operate and what are they?

Unveiling the Core of Chemical Peels

Chemical solutions are applied to the skin during chemical peels, causing the skin to exfoliate and finally peel off. Regenerated skin replaces the dead skin, and it is typically healthier and less wrinkled. A variety of cosmetic benefits are offered by the technique, which involves the controlled destruction of certain skin areas and tissue regeneration.

A Solution for Every Skin Type

Chemical peels are attractive because they may be customized to meet each patient's needs. There are many levels of peels, from mild to severe. Deep peels target more serious problems including precancerous growths while medium peels tackle acne scars and substantial pigmentation. Light peels address superficial wrinkles and uneven skin tone (*Soleymani et al., 2018*).

Your Candidacy for the Procedure

Sun damage, hyperpigmentation, fine wrinkles, and minor scarring are all conditions that chemical peels can improve. They aren't the best option for everyone, though. Alternative therapies could be necessary for those with particular skin types, health issues, or pharmaceutical regimens. You can be guided by a full consultation with a knowledgeable expert.

The Skin's Intermission: Prepping and Post-care

In order to prepare your skin for the peel, it may be necessary to do a skin evaluation and administer a preliminary treatment regimen. Aftercare is essential. You shouldn't go outside in the sun for a time because your skin will be extremely sensitive. You make a strict SPF regiment and a moisturizer your best buddies.

Let's Talk Dollars: The Cost Aspect

Chemical peels are typically not covered by insurance because they are an elective cosmetic procedure. The cost varies according to the clinic's standing, the intensity of the peel, and the patient's location. You could spend as little as $150 on mild peels, but severe peels can cost several thousand dollars.

The Ticking Clock: Longevity of Results

The results' resilience varies. Deep peels offer longer lasting remedies whereas light peels may need to be repeated every few weeks. Longevity is also influenced by lifestyle factors including sun exposure and skincare practices.

Chemical peels present a special chance to control the story of your skin by removing imperfections and exposing a revitalized layer beneath. Many people find the procedure to be an enticing alternative due to its adaptability, wide applicability, and possibility for transformation. Professional counseling is important because it comes with risks, just like any medical procedure. Depending on your decisions and commitments, this chapter in your skincare book may either be a passing page or leave a lasting impression.

PRP Therapy

Although Platelet-Rich Plasma (PRP) therapy is sometimes referred to as the "vampire facial," it is not a gimmick created by Hollywood. PRP therapy, a facet of regenerative medicine, uses your own blood's innate capacity for healing to hasten tissue regeneration and repair.

Unpacking the PRP Acronym

As the name implies, platelet-rich plasma is plasma that has a high concentration of platelets. Your blood contains platelets, which aid in blood clotting and wound healing. PRP is made by pulling a tiny amount of blood, separating the components with a centrifuge, and then removing the platelet-rich portion.

The How-To of PRP Therapy

PRP therapy is typically performed without hospitalization. The PRP is produced by taking a blood sample from you, typically from the arm. Your skin's targeted areas are then reinjected with this enriched plasma to promote the creation of natural collagen, skin tightening, and general rejuvenation. It's an intriguing idea to use one's own tissues to improve the functionality of another area of the body.

Tailoring the Treatment

PRP is unique due to its adaptability. In order to increase the efficacy of other therapies like microneedling or laser therapy, it is frequently combined with them. The neck, hands, and scalp are other possible treatment locations in addition to the face, where it is frequently utilized for facial rejuvenation. PRP has showed promise in reviving dormant hair follicles to treat hair loss (*Hasiba-Pappas et al., 2022*).

Who Should Consider PRP?

People who want to treat early aging symptoms, hair thinning, or even certain types of scarring are frequently candidates for PRP. However, those with skin disorders, certain cancers, or those taking particular drugs might need to think about alternative therapies. A healthcare professional should be consulted for a customized treatment plan.

The Post-Procedure Phase

Given that PRP therapy is non-invasive, recovery is often modest. It is normal to expect some swelling, bruising, or redness in the treatment region, but this normally goes away in a few days. After-treatment maintenance entails limiting sun exposure, applying a high-quality moisturizer, and wearing sunscreen.

Investment Breakdown

Several variables, including geographic location, practitioner skill, and if additional operations are being done concurrently, affect the price of PRP treatments. The cost of a session can range from $500 to $2,000, and for the best effects, several sessions could be required.

Results' Lifespan

In comparison to other non-invasive treatments, PRP therapy typically provides longer-lasting outcomes, especially when used for applications like hair regeneration. To maintain the advantages, maintenance sessions are typically advised.

PRP therapy uses your body's natural components to provide aesthetic treatments a new perspective. It is an attractive option for people in search of aesthetic perfection due to its versatile uses, little downtime, and potential for long-lasting results. However, customization and consultation are essential. To reap the advantages to the fullest extent, it is essential to customize the treatment to your unique needs and adhere to a rigorous post-care program.

Laser Hair Removal

Instead of temporary solutions like waxing, shaving, or threading, laser hair removal is becoming the standard. It's a cutting-edge answer to an age-old problem, relieving you of the monotony of regular grooming while also leaving you with the sleek, hairless look you've always wanted.

Understanding the Laser Lingo

'Laser' is an abbreviation for 'light amplification by stimulated emission of radiation,' which is what the technology actually does. In simple terms, it is a beam of light that has been sharply concentrated. The pigment in hair and skin known as melanin is the focus of hair removal lasers. Once the light energy has been absorbed by the melanin, it is transformed into heat, which harms the hair follicles over time and causes hair loss .

From Consultation to Calibration

A consultation is typically the initial stage in the laser hair removal process. During this time, your hair, skin, and any current medications will be discussed. Based on these variables, laser settings are calibrated to guarantee both safety and effectiveness. Patients are typically advised to stay out of the sun and avoid tanning in any way before treatment for the best outcomes.

The In-Office Experience

Depending on the treatment area, the operation can last anywhere from 20 minutes to an hour. Laser pulses are emitted by a portable device, and discomfort is reduced by a cooling mechanism or gel. Most people describe it as a "snapping" sensation against the skin, albeit it isn't completely pain-free.

Spotlight on Suitability

Although a variety of skin tones and hair types can benefit from laser hair removal, people with light complexion and dark hair typically see the best results. Darker skin tones might now benefit more from laser technology thanks to advancements in the field.

Post-Procedure Protocol

You can have some redness and swelling following the session that resembles a minor sunburn. These adverse effects usually disappear within a few days. Following therapy, it is strongly advised that patients use sunscreen and abstain from hot baths and excessive exercise for at least 24 hours.

Zooming in on Costs

The cost of laser hair removal is high. To remove all traces of hair, you'll need repeated treatments, which can cost anything from $50 for a tiny area like the upper lip to $300 for a bigger area like the back or legs. You should expect to make a large investment all in all.

The Long View

The benefits of laser hair removal are that they are semi-permanent. For the majority of people, hair growth is significantly reduced, and any hair that does regrowth is usually finer and lighter. In order to prevent undesired hair, periodic maintenance procedures may be required (*Vaidya et al., 2023*).

A high-tech, long-term answer to an ongoing issue is provided by laser hair removal. Although there are substantial upfront expenditures, the advantages—smooth skin, less time spent grooming, and an increase in confidence—make it a desirable choice for many. To verify you're an appropriate candidate for the treatment, conduct your research and speak with a recognized professional.

Cellulite Treatment

Cellulite, also referred to as "orange peel skin," has long baffled people who strive for an attractive appearance. The majority of the dimpled skin may be found on the thighs, buttocks, and even the abdomen, which frequently prompts people to look into different treatments to smooth things out.

What is Cellulite?

Skin conditions like cellulite have a lumpy, uneven appearance. It's not a sign of any underlying health problems, but for many people, it may be an aesthetic worry. Basically, the uneven texture is caused when fat cells press on the skin and fibrous bands pull the skin down.

Types of Treatments

There are numerous surgical and non-surgical treatments available to address cellulite. The goal of non-invasive procedures including radiofrequency, laser, and acoustic wave therapy is to dissolve the fibrous bands and promote the formation of collagen. Cellfina and Cellulaze are invasive procedures that target structural problems under the skin (*Gabriel et al., 2023*).

Non-Surgical Routes: How They Work

Consider radiofrequency (RF) as an illustration. By heating the skin's deeper layers, RF energy encourages the creation of collagen and improves the texture of the skin. It's a quick, office-based treatment that may be finished with no downtime in an hour or two.

Invasive Treatments: Going Under the Knife

Small incisions are made to remove the fibrous bands producing the dimples in surgical treatments like Cellfina for individuals who would want a more immediate solution. The effects can persist for up to three years, but keep in mind that there are dangers associated with surgery, such as infection and scars.

Who's the Best Candidate?

The majority of people are not good candidates for cellulite therapy. The effectiveness of therapies can vary depending on your cellulite severity, general health, and lifestyle choices. To receive a personalized evaluation based on your unique needs, speak with a trained medical professional.

The Price of Perfection: What Will It Cost?

Depending on the region and the technology employed, non-surgical treatments might cost anywhere from $500 to $4,000. Prices for surgical procedures like Cellfina start at roughly $5,000, so they might cost a little more. It's critical to balance the expense with the predicted durability and effectiveness of the outcomes.

A Realistic Perspective: What to Expect

When considering therapy for cellulite, it's crucial to have reasonable expectations. While most treatments can dramatically lessen cellulite's appearance, they might not always be successful. Diet, exercise, and hydration are other lifestyle aspects that affect how long your effects last.

The advancements in cosmetic medicine have made treating cellulite more feasible than ever. The secret is to seek advice from a licensed healthcare professional to determine which course of action will be most beneficial for your particular circumstance. Understanding your options and acting wisely are the first steps to smoother, more confident skin, whether you decide for a DIY cream or a more sophisticated procedure.

RF Microneedling

Microneedling and radiofrequency are two extremely potent cosmetic treatments, and when they are combined, you get RF Microneedling, which is known for its ability to tighten skin and stimulate collagen. The method has been making waves in the dermatology community and is frequently praised for its versatility in treating a variety of skin conditions. There seems to be very little that this treatment can't manage, from fine lines and acne scars to slack skin and big pores.

Understanding the Procedure

The dual-action treatment is at the heart of RF Microneedling. Depending on the problem being treated, microneedles only penetrate the skin so far before producing controlled harm. The radiofrequency radiation released heats the skin's deeper layers while the body shifts into repair mode. The components of young, firm skin, collagen and elastin, are produced more readily as a result of this heat (*Kornstein, 2020*).

Setting it Apart from Standard Microneedling

Although conventional microneedling also claims to rejuvenate skin by inflicting micro-injuries that spur the creation of collagen, the use of radiofrequency raises the procedure to new heights. The RF radiation provides a more controlled and targeted form of treatment, allowing you to target the deeper layers of skin without affecting the top layer, producing quicker and more obvious results.

Who Should Consider It?

RF Microneedling is a flexible procedure that works on a variety of skin types and tones. It works particularly well for people who have problems with scars, sagging skin, or skin laxity brought on by aging. A licensed dermatologist should be consulted to determine if this treatment is appropriate for your skin type and condition.

What's the Downtime?

Because RF Microneedling is so minimally invasive, recovery time is typically relatively short. Common but transient adverse effects include mild redness, swelling, or a sunburn-like sensation. Most individuals can get back to their normal routines in a day or two, but it's crucial to avoid vigorous exercise and direct sunlight for about a week.

The Financial Angle

There is some financial outlay need to invest in RF Microneedling. Depending on the patient's location, the provider's level of experience, and the particular problems being addressed, the cost of treatment may change. Prices typically range from $500 to $1,500 each session, with numerous sessions frequently necessary for the best outcomes.

RF Microneedling is an intriguing point of confluence between biology and technology in the developing field of cosmetic dermatology. It claims to balance the scales between invasiveness and outcomes, providing a non-surgical yet effective solution for a variety of skin issues. This might be the procedure you've been looking for if you're prepared to make a bold move toward improved skin quality without having surgery.

CHAPTER SEVEN

7. *Plastic Surgery FAQs*

Plastic surgery can change your life, but it's normal to have doubts and worries before making the decision. What distinguishes plastic surgery for cosmetic and reconstructive purposes? How can you determine whether you'd be a good candidate for a certain procedure? What qualities need to a plastic surgeon have? These are just a few of the questions that people regularly ask, which we'll answer in this chapter.

The most popular plastic surgery procedures, potential risks and complications, healing times, and financial factors will all be covered. We want to arm you with all the knowledge you need to make informed decisions about your plastic surgery experience. You'll know what to anticipate and feel confident about your abilities to know more about the plastic surgery industry by the end of this chapter.

What is the Difference Between Cosmetic and Reconstructive Plastic Surgery?

Many people are perplexed by the subtleties of plastic surgery because the art and science of it are frequently enmeshed in a tangle of truths and myths. Making the distinction between cosmetic and reconstructive plastic surgery is one of the most frequent sources of confusion.

Cosmetic Surgery: The Aesthetic Approach

The goal of cosmetic surgery is to improve your appearance. Here, we're talking about elective treatments, which you choose to have done for aesthetic purposes only rather than to improve particular physical or facial characteristics. This includes operations like liposuction, facelifts, and breast augmentation.

Reconstructive Surgery: The Functional Fix

Reconstructive surgery, on the other hand, has its roots in a need for treatment. The objective is to correct disfigurement brought on by burns, trauma, congenital deformities, or disease, as well as to restore function. Consider sophisticated skin grafting for burn sufferers, cleft lip restoration, breast reconstruction following a mastectomy, etc.

The Diverging Roads

So even though plastic surgeons manipulate tissues during both reconstructive and cosmetic procedures, their goals are different. A branch of the larger field of plastic surgery is called cosmetic surgery. In contrast to cosmetic surgery, which is frequently thought of as the core of plastic surgery, reconstructive surgery is frequently covered by health insurance due to its medical need.

What Are the Most Common Plastic Surgery Procedures?

Plastic surgery has entered the lives of regular people, moving beyond the world of Hollywood's elite. But which operations do people typically choose? Let's sort through the most in demand.

Breast Augmentation

This surgical surgery tries to augment breast size or replace breast volume that has been lost as a result of pregnancy, weight loss, or aging. The most popular techniques are fat grafting or implanting.

Liposuction

Excess fat removal surgery can be performed on problem areas such the stomach, thighs, and buttocks.

Rhinoplasty

This procedure, also known as a "nose job," modifies the nose's size or form to better balance it with the rest of the face.

Tummy Tuck

In a procedure known as an abdominoplasty, the abdominal muscles are tightened and extra skin is removed to create a smoother, tighter abdomen.

Eyelid Surgery

This operation, called blepharoplasty, improves bags and puffiness under the eyes as well as sagging or drooping eyelids.

Botox and Fillers

Despite not requiring surgery, these injectable procedures are frequently brought up in discussions about cosmetic surgery since they can temporarily address facial volume loss and wrinkles.

Hair Transplant

This technique, which is becoming more popular, is most popular among men and involves moving hair follicles from one area of the body to the scalp.

Brazilian Butt Lift (BBL)

By moving fat from other body areas, this technique improves the size and form of the buttocks.

Facelift

This surgical treatment, known as rhytidectomy in the medical community, is used to restore a more youthful appearance by tightening excess skin on the face and neck.

Before choosing a technique, it is crucial to thoroughly investigate the dangers and benefits that each one presents. With the proper information, you are empowered to make decisions that are in line with your aesthetic objectives and health considerations.

Am I a Good Candidate for Plastic Surgery?

You're interested in plastic surgery, maybe even excited about it, but the major question is: Are you a good candidate? The solution is not a one-size-fits-all formula but a concoction of several elements customized to your particular profile. You can read more about what qualifies you for plastic surgery below.

Physical Health

A healthy body serves as the foundation for any surgery that succeeds. You need to be in good health overall to have the best results and the fewest possible complications. Your surgical procedure could be complicated, and recovery could be difficult, if you have illnesses like diabetes, hypertension, or a weakened immune system.

Psychological Wellness

Unbelievably, how you're feeling and thinking matters a great deal. A satisfactory result can be created by having a good view, reasonable expectations, and a steady frame of mind. People who seek surgical solutions for pervasive emotional or psychological problems may be on the wrong track.

Skin Quality

Ever wonder what your skin has to do with any of this? When skin stretching is included in operations like facelifts or tummy tucks, elastic, flexible skin typically responds better. On the other hand, skin that is thin or injured could not look its best.

Lifestyle Choices

Pre- and post-surgery, you might need to say goodbye to some routines and way of life decisions. For example, smoking can slow healing whereas a diet high in particular nutrients can hasten it. How prepared are you to make such lifestyle changes?

Financial Readiness

Particularly cosmetic surgeries that are not covered by insurance, surgeries can be expensive. Have you planned financially for post-operative care, medication, and potential lost wages?

Individual Goals

Different methods meet various needs. A breast lift might be a better option if your concern is sagging rather than enhanced body proportions, which breast augmentation may be ideal for. Talk freely with your surgeon about your aesthetic objectives; a skilled surgeon will be a helpful guide and an attentive listener.

Long-term Commitment

Although many surgical procedures produce long-lasting benefits, lifelong assurances are rare. Aging is unavoidable, and some operations might even need changes in the future. Are you prepared to make that dedication?

It takes more than just identifying a problem area and making an appointment to be a suitable candidate for plastic surgery. It entails a thorough assessment of your lifestyle, thoughts, and health. To determine whether you are a good candidate for the selected surgery, make sure you have a comprehensive consultation with a board-certified plastic surgeon. To become the best version of yourself, your surgeon and you both share the same objective. As a result, arrive prepared, make inquiries, and, most importantly, pay attention to your body and thoughts.

What Should I Look for in a Plastic Surgeon?

Similar to choosing an architect for your dream home, finding the best plastic surgeon is important. Your wellbeing and physical appearance are on the line, thus the stakes are high. Medical credentials are a must, but there are other minor factors that might have a big impact on how well your plastic surgery journey goes.

Board Certification

Plastic surgery board certification is a requirement for your potential surgeon. This guarantees they've undergone demanding training and fulfilled demanding requirements, proving proficiency in their industry. You should accept it as the absolute least; any less puts your safety in jeopardy.

Specialization

A general plastic surgeon may do a variety of operations, but if you're interested in a particular procedure, such as rhinoplasty or a Brazilian Butt Lift, it's best to select one performed by a surgeon who specializes in that field. With significant experience comes specialization, which produces better honed abilities.

Reviews and Reputation

What have other people said about the surgeon you're considering? Investigate third-party review sites in addition to the patient testimonials on the doctor's website. Asking those who have undergone similar treatments for recommendations is another option. Although every person's experiences are unique, trends in pleasure or dissatisfaction can offer important insights.

Before and After Photos

This image collection may provide a wealth of knowledge. Are the outcomes appearing naturally? Do they match your aesthetic objectives? Pay close attention to patients with similar face or bodily features to yours. These images might provide some insight into the surgeon's personality and skills.

Consultation Experience

Not only does the surgeon examine you during the initial appointment, but you also have a chance to evaluate them. Is the surgeon attentive to your worries and providing tailored remedies? Are the dangers and problems disclosed? The best surgeon may not be the one who rushes you through the consultation.

Hospital Privileges

A encouraging sign is if your surgeon has privileges at reputable hospitals, even if your treatment is an outpatient one. This typically means they have undergone peer review to ensure they are competent and uphold certain moral and ethical standards.

Cost

While it may be tempting to shop around, keep in mind that this is an investment in yourself rather than a purchase. Unreasonably low costs could be a sign of a compromised product's quality or additional expenses. Always double-check that the offered price covers all expected expenditures, such as those associated with the anesthesiologist, the surgery center, and any necessary follow-up treatment.

Postoperative Care

Ask about the recovery schedule. Who will oversee your post-care, and how easily can you reach them for follow-up appointments? This is an important factor to take into account because thorough aftercare is essential for reducing risks and problems.

Your ideal plastic surgeon should be a skilled expert whose mindset meshes with yours and who also adheres to your medical and aesthetic needs. It's a fine line to walk, but it's important to make sure you put your health and your goals in qualified hands.

What Are the Risks Associated With Plastic Surgery?

It's critical to balance the benefits and drawbacks of a laser or surgical procedure. Plastic surgery certainly has the power to alter, providing newfound self-confidence and physical benefits, but it is not without its drawbacks. When it comes to surgical procedures, ignorance is not bliss; rather, it could put one's life in jeopardy.

Anesthesia Complications

While the majority of patients concentrate on the process itself, anesthesia, which is frequently used to make procedures more comfortable, has its own set of dangers. From mild symptoms like lightheadedness and nausea to more serious ones like allergic responses or respiratory problems. These hazards can be reduced but not totally eliminated by a skilled anesthesiologist and a thorough pre-surgery evaluation.

Infections

Every surgical operation carries some risk of infection. Antibiotics and sanitized facilities aid in reducing this hazard, but there is always a slight possibility that germs will still manage to enter, slowing down your recovery and possibly leading to more severe consequences.

Bleeding and Hematoma

Hematoma is a disorder characterized by a pocket of blood resembling a huge, painful bruise; while some bleeding is expected following surgery, excessive bleeding can lead to hematoma. In rare circumstances, a different treatment may be required to drain the gathered blood.

Scarring

Ironically, plastic surgery leaves scars as a reminder of its failure to improve a person's appearance. Although doctors do their best to prevent scarring, even the most careful patient may be left with a discolored or elevated scar despite their best efforts.

Nerve Damage

Nerve injury is a risk that comes with various procedures. In severe situations, symptoms like paralysis can range from slight tingling and numbness to more serious problems. You should first have a thorough conversation with your physician about this possibility.

Surgical Errors

Despite years of intensive training, surgeons are nevertheless human and prone to mistakes. Asymmetry, tissue loss, or even more serious consequences necessitating several corrective procedures are all possible outcomes of major surgical errors.

Emotional Toll

It's critical to keep in mind that plastic surgery can significantly affect your emotional state in addition to changing your physical appearance. Unrealistic expectations might result in post-operative disappointment that can take the form of regret, melancholy, or anxiety.

Long-Term Complications

Some operations, especially those involving implants, can need for follow-up surgery. Additionally, as you age, your body gradually changes, which could result in issues or unhappiness years after the first operation.

Financial Strain

The cost of excellent plastic surgery is high. The financial load can be a stressor that affects your mental health, especially when combined with prospective expenses for post-operative care or, in the worst cases, corrective surgery.

Be a knowledgeable shopper. Consult with many experts, research the topic yourself if you can, and study relevant scientific papers. Your body is what it is. Understanding the plastic surgery industry's pros and cons is essential to making an educated decision.

What is the Recovery Period of Different Plastic Surgery Procedures?

If you're thinking about having any kind of plastic surgery, you've probably wondered what the recovery period will be like. How soon will you be able to resume your regular schedule, obligations at work, and social activities? Recovery time is a health issue as well as a logistical one. Longer recuperation times frequently indicate more extensive operations, which have additional factors to take into account.

Breast Augmentation

A week off work is typically required for breast augmentation. You must wait about a month before returning to rigorous exercise, though. Following your surgeon's instructions is essential to preventing issues like implant displacement.

Tummy Tuck: The Long Haul

In general, recovery from tummy tucks takes two to three weeks, and there is a longer period of downtime afterward. But before you can fully participate in all of your usual activities, it could take up to two months.

Brazilian Butt Lift (BBL): Sit with Caution

It may take up to eight weeks until you are totally able to sit without a BBL-specific cushion, so you should avoid sitting directly on your buttocks for at least two weeks.

Liposuction: It Varies

Today's less invasive procedures allow for modest liposuction recovery times of just a few days. More involved operations, however, can take a few weeks.

Rhinoplasty: A Nose by Any Other Name

A nasal splint must be worn for at least a week after a rhinoplasty, during which time you must recover. Expect some modest swelling for a few weeks even after the splint is taken off.

Hair Transplant: Not a Quick Fix

Even though you might return to work in a few days, the changes to your scalp, bruising, and swelling could last for up to two weeks.

Eyelid Surgery: Keep Those Eyes Closed

The majority of patients recover from eyelid surgery within ten days, although for a few weeks afterward, your eyes may be sensitive to light and appear bruised.

Chemical Peels: Surface vs Deep

A minor peel may just require a few days to recover from, whereas a thorough peel may take two weeks or longer and cause redness to last for months.

Abdominal Etching: Quicker than You'd Think

In most cases, patients can resume their usual exercise routine within a month and go back to work within a week.

PRP Therapy: Almost Instant

Most patients can continue their regular activities right away after receiving platelet-rich plasma treatment because there is typically little downtime.

The recovery period you'll experience will seem insignificant in comparison to the potential long-term advantages of a successful surgery. But be ready for these essential breaks in your routine. It's not only about getting better; it's also about getting the most out of the money you put in yourself. To ensure the smoothest recovery possible, your surgeon will provide you with a specific recovery plan.

How Long Do the Results Last for Each Procedure?

Plastic surgery outcomes can be life-altering, but they frequently have a sort of shelf life. The duration of these alterations varies depending on the surgery and your body's particular reaction to it.

Breast Augmentation: A Decade or More

Implants made of silicone and saline often last 10 to 20 years. They are not, however, perpetual devices. To replace outdated implants or to change their size and contour, many women choose revision operations.

Tummy Tuck: A Lifelong Commitment

Although the benefits are thought to be permanent, large weight changes can change the results. For effects that last, maintaining a constant weight is essential.

Brazilian Butt Lift (BBL): Long-lasting but Not Forever

Since BBL utilizes your body's fat, the results might last for many years. The duration of the outcomes will, inevitably, be impacted by aging and weight fluctuations.

Liposuction: Permanent Fat Removal, Conditional Results

The fat cells that liposuction removes are permanently gone. But gaining weight might cause new fat cells to form, changing the contour of your body.

Rhinoplasty: Nearly Permanent

Unless you suffer a serious injury to the area, the effects of a rhinoplasty are thought to be permanent. Aging might still bring about subtle changes.

Hair Transplant: Differing Durabilities

While natural, non-transplanted hair may continue to fall out and require treatments in the future, transplanted hair is typically permanent.

Eyelid Surgery: A Decade of Youthful Eyes

The effects of eyelid surgery can persist for up to ten years, but they won't reverse the effects of aging naturally. As they get older, some people choose to have revision surgery.

Chemical Peels: From Months to Years

While the effects of deeper peels can linger for years, lighter peels may only last a few months. These effects may last longer with additional treatments.

Abdominal Etching: Years with Caveats

The outcomes are comparatively permanent, much like liposuction, however weight gain might ruin the sculpted aesthetic.

PRP Therapy: Highly Variable

The duration of PRP therapy varies depending on the treatment region and the patient, frequently necessitating routine maintenance sessions.

Facelift: Up to a Decade

Although facelifts can turn the hands of time back up to ten years, aging never stops. To keep their results, many people choose to make tiny adjustments.

Botox and Fillers: Temporary Satisfaction

Depending on the type and location treated, these treatments might last anywhere from three months to two years. Regular maintenance is crucial.

Planning your plastic surgery journey requires having a clear understanding of how long you can anticipate the results to last. It affects not only your decision to proceed with the surgery but also how you prepare for the future in terms of your life and finances. You can take a calculated step toward long-lasting aesthetic satisfaction by combining the understanding of expected longevity with a surgeon's abilities.

What Plastic Surgery Procedures Leave Permanent Scars?

Anyone thinking about getting plastic surgery typically worries about the possibility of having lasting scars. There are always incisions after surgery, and there is always a scar. These scars are unavoidable, but their severity and longevity depend on many factors, including the nature of the treatment, your skin, and the expertise of the surgeon.

Unavoidable But Hidden: Tummy Tuck

The scar after a stomach tuck is typically located low on the abdomen so that it can be hidden by undergarments or a bathing suit. The scar may lighten with time, but it will never disappear entirely.

Breast Augmentation and Lift: Scars With Options

The areola, the breast fold, and the armpit are all possible sites for scarring after breast surgery. These scars are permanent even though they eventually vanish.

Rhinoplasty: Minimal but Present

The tissue that separates your nostrils, known as the columella, will be scarred slightly if you opt for open rhinoplasty. Since incisions are made inside the nostrils, closed rhinoplasty does not leave noticeable scarring.

Facelift: Craftily Concealed

Scars following a facelift typically begin in the lower scalp and extend from the temples. These are intended to be discrete and are frequently covered by the natural features of the face and hair.

Hair Transplant: Tiny Dots or a Line

Small, circular scars will be spread out across the donor area with Follicular Unit Extraction (FUE), while a long, thin scar will be left behind with Follicular Unit Transplantation (FUT).

Liposuction: Small But Permanent

Although liposuction incisions are often small and positioned carefully, they do leave behind scars that cannot be removed.

However, they are simple to hide due to their size and placement.

Brazilian Butt Lift: Nearly Invisible

The scars left behind by a BBL are often relatively minor and gradually lighten with time. Additionally, they are placed carefully to blend in as little as possible.

Cleft Lip and Palate Repair: Unavoidable but Improved

Although there is a scar from this reconstructive surgery, expert surgeons can decrease its look with additional surgeries.

Scar Revision: Irony of Sorts

A new scar will be formed throughout the treatment even though the goal of scar revision is to lessen the visibility of existing scars. The new scar, however, normally looks considerably less prominent.

Burn Reconstruction: Scars Changing Scars

While scarring is inevitable following skin grafts and other forms of reconstructive surgery, the goal is to replace extensive scarring with something less obvious.

There are other factors besides the surgery itself that can affect whether a procedure leaves a noticeable, permanent scar. Scarring can also be influenced by factors like your skin type, age, and how well you adhere to post-operative care instructions. Improved outcomes for a variety of surgeries are now possible thanks to continually developing advanced surgical methods and scar management therapies. Knowing what kind of scarring to expect from your selected surgery will help you set reasonable expectations and get ready for the recovery process.

How Much Does Plastic Surgery Cost Depending on the Procedure?

It's impossible to avoid debating plastic surgery's financial commitment, but it's also fascinating to do so. The total price of a surgery is more than the sum of its parts, which might include anything from the surgeon's fee to the cost of the hospital stay, anesthesia, and follow-up care. Don't forget the geography also; pricing might vary greatly depending on where you are. But since you're here for the numbers, let's break down the prices for a few common practices.

Tummy Tuck

Typically, a belly tuck costs between $5,000 and $10,000. If you're thinking of combining it with liposuction or other operations, the cost can increase.

Breast Augmentation

The price of the procedure can range from $6,000 to $12,000. Silicone implants are often more expensive than saline implants.

Rhinoplasty

A nose operation can cost between $5,000 and $10,000, or even more if major structural alterations are required.

Facelift

Facelift prices typically range from $7,000 to $15,000, depending on the techniques used and the amount of the lift.

Hair Transplant

The price mostly depends on how many grafts you require. You're looking at an average price range of $4,000 to $15,000.

Liposuction

Each component of the body has a different price. Liposuction typically costs between $2,000 and $8,000 per treated region.

Brazilian Butt Lift

Depending on your region and particular needs, a BBL will typically cost between $4,000 and $12,000.

Cleft Lip and Palate Repair

Even though insurance frequently pays for this, the out-of-pocket expense without insurance might be anywhere between $5,000 and $10,000.

Scar Revision

Depending on the amount of the rewrite and whether alternative methods are used, budget between $1,000 and $4,000.

Burn Reconstruction

The cost is highly variable because this typically involves several procedures spread out over time, but in extreme circumstances, it can potentially exceed $100,000.

Botox and Fillers

While fillers can cost anywhere from $600 to $2,000 per syringe, botox typically ranges from $200 to $600 per session.

Why then do prices range so widely? Each procedure is developed specifically for the patient. The figures can change depending on the procedure's intricacy, the surgeon's experience, and the facility where it is carried out. Additional expenses include follow-up visits, prescriptions, and occasionally corrective operations. Get a thorough overview of all prices up front to ensure there are no unforeseen expenses impeding your path to aesthetic fulfillment.

Can I Undergo Plastic Surgery if I Have a Pre-existing Medical Condition?

It takes a high level of caution, planning, and knowledge to go through a procedure if you already pre-existing medical issues and want to go through plastic surgery procedure. Although it's not a formal no-go zone, consider it a region that needs clear signage. Safety is the main issue here, both during and after the surgery.

Medical Evaluation

A complete medical evaluation is a requirement before considering any particular operations. Your primary care physician and other specialists should work closely with your plastic surgeon. Depending on your illness, you might anticipate a range of tests, such as blood testing, heart screening, and possibly even diagnostic imaging.

Chronic Conditions

Under the direction of their specialized doctors, patients with diabetes, heart ailments, or pulmonary problems must stabilize these diseases. For example, uncontrolled diabetes can significantly impede wound healing and increase the risk of infections.

Weight Concerns

You might need to lose weight before surgery if you have a disease like obesity or metabolic syndrome. Excess weight can put more strain on your heart and lungs during surgery and increase surgical risks like blood clots.

Medication Adjustments

Long-term medicine is required for some diseases, which could have an impact on your operation or recuperation. Blood thinners, particular anti-seizure drugs, and a few over-the-counter vitamins might need to be modified or temporarily stopped.

Mental Health

Disorders like depression, anxiety, or other mood disorders can have an impact on both your preoperative preparation and postoperative recovery. When considering surgery, both physical and emotional wellness are essential.

Minor Conditions

It is typically less of an issue to have conditions like well-controlled hypothyroidism, stable asthma, or well-controlled blood pressure. Even though you still need a medical okay, getting surgery is frequently a simpler process.

Financial Considerations

Contrary to popular belief, your pre-existing ailment may result in greater prices. Your final bill may increase if you need longer hospital stays, more tests, or expert consultations.

Final Clearance

The final approval is granted when the plastic surgeon and all of your other medical professionals agree that the advantages outweigh the drawbacks. Once you've been given the all-clear, your surgical team will endeavor to optimize every aspect for the best result.

You are not immediately disqualified from the life-changing experience of plastic surgery because of a pre-existing condition. The trade-off is that you'll have to make your way through a more complicated pre-operative maze, armed with a library of medical knowledge and a team of healthcare professionals at your side at all times.

Conclusion

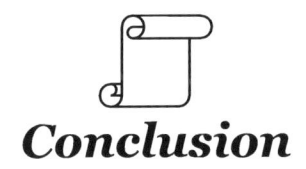

Now that our journey through the many facets of the field of plastic surgery has come to a close, let's take a moment to reflect on what we've learned. We have journeyed through history, investigated the techniques, and considered the benefits and drawbacks of many approaches. With a strong foundation for decision-making, this book aims to be a one-stop shop for anyone thinking about a journey into cosmetic or reconstructive upgrades.

Beginning with the fundamentals, we clarified what plastic surgery entails while briefly discussing its historical foundations, which show that it is not merely a manifestation of the current era but rather a practice with a long history in humankind. We investigated the factors that influence people to think about having plastic surgery, busting myths and giving you an accurate picture of the prices, advantages, and risks.

For women, many operations were explored, including Brazilian butt lifts, laser treatments, and breast augmentation, each of which offered a distinctive type of metamorphosis. Men are increasingly exploring the field of cosmetic modifications, so we broke down the subtleties of procedures like hair transplants, belly etching, and jawline upgrades for them.

Beyond the promise of aesthetic enhancement, reconstructive surgery serves as a reminder that there is a field devoted to treating deformities, mending scars, and even providing post-cancer remedies like breast reconstruction. These treatments not only revitalize the body but also the spirit, frequently offering patients a second opportunity at living a "normal" life.

Another key rest stop on our journey was aesthetic dermatology, which provided less intrusive alternatives for individuals who weren't yet ready for surgery. These procedures, which range from mole removal to PRP therapy, can be both preventive and remedial, enabling patients to take charge of the condition and appearance of their skin.

Our journey through this maze naturally raised questions. Our FAQ section sought to foresee and address problems, including topics like candidacy, recuperation, and even debunking widely held myths. Before making a decision this important in your life, it's important to be both eager and knowledgeable.

Another unavoidable concern was cost. It can be tempting to ignore the financial investment and concentrate entirely on how transformative plastic surgery can be. Some procedures might be covered by insurance, but it's important to enter this situation well aware of the associated financial commitments.

The idea of empowerment via knowledge has been the main theme throughout. Every action, every decision has its own inherent set of potentials and constraints. Your pleasure with the outcome might be considerably impacted by being aware of these.

You should keep in mind that the purpose of this book is not to promote or criticize plastic surgery, but rather to provide you with the information you need to make an informed decision. You made the decision, it was your body, and hopefully now you can see it with a more enlightened perspective.

Thank you for sticking with us on this educational journey. May you find this book to be a trustworthy guide as you decide whether to get plastic surgery.

Your Opinion Matters

Did this book help you in some way?
If so, we'd love to hear about it!
Scan the QR code below to leave your honest review.

Scan here!

About The Author

Dr. Samantha Reynolds is a clinical dermatologist and surgeon. Her fields of practice include dermatology, plastic surgery, facial sculpting, and body contouring.
Dr. Reynolds is known for her attention to detail and her commitment to providing personalized care to each of her patients. She believes in a holistic approach to plastic surgery, considering not only the physical aspects but also the emotional well-being of her patients.

Beyond her practice, Dr. Reynolds is actively involved in medical research and education. Her contributions to medical journals and conferences have earned her respect and recognition among her peers. In addition to her medical endeavors, Dr. Reynolds volunteers her time to organizations that support individuals on their journey to self-healing from childhood trauma and abuse.

References

1. Singh, V. (2017, June 8). *"Sushruta: The father of surgery."* PubMed Central (PMC). https://doi.org/10.4103/njms.NJMS_33_17
2. Development of Plastic Surgery - PubMed. (2015, June 1). https://doi.org/10.2298/mpns1506199p
3. MBBS, R. C. (2018, July 17). *"Can breast reduction surgery relieve back pain? Can Breast Reduction Surgery Relieve Back Pain?"* | Ohio State Medical Center. https://wexnermedical.osu.edu/blog/can-breast-reduction-surgery-relieve-back-pain
4. Ri, C., Yu, J., Mao, J., & Zhao, M. (2022, June 2). *"Trends in Breast Augmentation Research: A Bibliometric Analysis - Aesthetic Plastic Surgery."* SpringerLink. https://doi.org/10.1007/s00266-022-02904-9
5. Stevens, W. G., Stoker, D. A., Freeman, M. E., Quardt, S. M., & Hirsch, E. M. (2007, March 1). *"Mastopexy Revisited: A Review of 150 Consecutive Cases for Complication and Revision Rates."* OUP Academic. https://doi.org/10.1016/j.asj.2006.12.014
6. "A Journey Through Liposuction and Liposculture: Review," ScienceDirect. https://doi.org/10.1016/j.amsu.2017.10.024
7. Regan, J. P., & Casaubon, J. T. (2023, July 24). Abdominoplasty - StatPearls - NCBI Bookshelf. https://www.ncbi.nlm.nih.gov/books/NBK431058/
8. "Brazilian Butt Lift" Performed by Board-Certified Brazilian Plastic Surgeons: Reports of an Expert Opinion Survey - PubMed. (2019, September 1). https://doi.org/10.1097/PRS.0000000000006020
9. Sanan, A., & Most, S. P. (2021, March 2). Rhytidectomy (Face-Lift Surgery). Rhytidectomy (Face-Lift Surgery) |

Brow, Face, Forehead Lift | JAMA | JAMA Network. https://doi.org/10.1001/jama.2018.17292

10. Zhu, X., Zhang, B., & Huang, Y. (2022, October 31). *"Trends of rhinoplasty research in the last decade with bibliometric analysis."* Frontiers. https://doi.org/10.3389/fsurg.2022.1067934

11. Naik, M. N., Honavar, S. G., Das, S., Desai, S., & Dhepe, N. (2009, June 2). *"Blepharoplasty: An Overview."* PubMed Central (PMC). https://doi.org/10.4103/0974-2077.53092

12. *"Lip Augmentation: Background, History of the Procedure, Problem."* (2023, January 18). https://emedicine.medscape.com/article/1288367-overview

13. Sadick, N. S., & Palmisano, L. (2009, May 1). *"Cheek Augmentation With Dermicol-P35 27G."* OUP Academic. https://doi.org/10.1016/j.asj.2009.03.004

14. Fink, B., & Prager, M. (2014, January 7). *"The Effect of Incobotulinumtoxin A and Dermal Filler Treatment on Perception of Age, Health, and Attractiveness of Female Faces."* PubMed Central (PMC). Retrieved September 13, 2023, from https://www.ncbi.nlm.nih.gov/pmc/articles/PMC3930539/

15. Khalkhal, E., Rezaei-Tavirani, M., Zali, M. R., & Akbari, Z. (2019, December 1). *"The Evaluation of Laser Application in Surgery: A Review Article."* PubMed Central (PMC). https://doi.org/10.15171/jlms.2019.S18

16. Somogyi, R. B., Ziolkowski, N., Osman, F., Ginty, A., & Brown, M. (2018, June 6). *"Breast reconstruction: Updated overview for primary care physicians."* PubMed Central (PMC). Retrieved September 13, 2023, from https://www.ncbi.nlm.nih.gov/pmc/articles/PMC5999246/

17. *"Plastic Surgery for Cleft Palate: Cleft Palate, Cleft Palate Appearance, How Does Cleft Palate Affect Hearing and Speech?"* (2019, May

20). https://emedicine.medscape.com/article/1280866-overview
18. Ogawa, R. (2019, March 1). *"Surgery for scar revision and reduction: from primary closure to flap surgery - Burns & Trauma."* BioMed Central. https://doi.org/10.1186/s41038-019-0144-5
19. Barret, J. P. (2004, July 31). *"ABC of burns: Burns reconstruction."* PubMed Central (PMC). https://doi.org/10.1136/bmj.329.7460.274
20. Barbara, G., Facchin, F., Buggio, L., Alberico, D., Frattaruolo, M. P., & Kustermann, A. (2017, July 21). *"Vaginal rejuvenation: current perspectives."* PubMed Central (PMC). https://doi.org/10.2147/IJWH.S99700
21. Tzolova, N., & Hadjiiski, O. (2008, March 31). *"Tissue Expansion Used as a Method of Reconstructive Surgery in Childhood."* PubMed Central (PMC). https://www.ncbi.nlm.nih.gov/pmc/articles/PMC3188126/
22. Vogel, J. E., Jimenez, F., Cole, J., Keene, S. A., Harris, J. A., Barrera, A., & Rose, P. T. (2013, January 1). *"Hair Restoration Surgery: The State of the Art."* OUP Academic. https://doi.org/10.1177/1090820X12468314
23. Sistemas e Publicações, G., & Viaro, M. (2019). RBCP - Abdominal etching. https://doi.org/10.5935/2177-1235.2019RBCP0205
24. Harris, W. C., & Raggio, B. S. (2022, May 1). *"Facial Chin Augmentation,"* StatPearls - NCBI Bookshelf. https://www.ncbi.nlm.nih.gov/books/NBK554506/
25. Benito-Ruiz, J., Raigosa, J. M., Manzano-Surroca, M., & Salvador, L. (2007, August 5). *"Male Chest Enhancement: Pectoral Implants - Aesthetic Plastic Surgery."* SpringerLink. https://doi.org/10.1007/s00266-007-9018-5
26. Saad, A. N., Arbelaez, J. P., & Benito, J. D. (2020, March 1). *"High Definition Liposculpture in Male Patients Using Reciprocating Power-Assisted Liposuction Technology:*

Techniques and Results in a Prospective Study." OUP Academic. https://doi.org/10.1093/asj/sjz218

27. Littara, A., Melone, R., Morales-Medina, J. C., Iannitti, T., & Palmieri, B. (2019, April 19). *"Cosmetic penile enhancement surgery: a 3-year single-centre retrospective clinical evaluation of 355 cases."* PubMed Central (PMC). https://doi.org/10.1038/s41598-019-41652-w

28. Holzmer, S. W., Lewis, P. G., Landau, M. J., & Hill, M. E. (2020, October 29). *"Surgical Management of Gynecomastia: A Comprehensive Review of the Literature."* PubMed Central (PMC). https://doi.org/10.1097/GOX.0000000000003161

29. Lem, M., Pham, J. T., Kim, J. K., & Tang, C. J. (2023, May 16). *"Changing Aesthetic Surgery Interest in Men: An 18-Year Analysis."* PubMed Central (PMC). https://doi.org/10.1007/s00266-023-03344-9

30. *"Laser Hair Removal Risks and Safety."* (2023). American Society of Plastic Surgeons. Retrieved September 13, 2023, from https://www.plasticsurgery.org/cosmetic-procedures/laser-hair-removal/safety

31. *"Plastic Surgery for Gynecomastia: Practice Essentials, History of the Procedure,"* (2023, June 6). https://emedicine.medscape.com/article/1273437-overview

32. Garg, S., Dahiya, N., & Gupta, S. (2014, March 7). *"Surgical Scar Revision: An Overview."* PubMed Central (PMC). https://doi.org/10.4103/0974-2077.129959

33. Klein, M. B., Donelan, M. B., & Spence, R. J. (2007, August 1). *"Reconstructive Surgery."* OUP Academic. https://doi.org/10.1097/BCR.0B013E318093E4A4

34. Sadaka, M. S., & Bakr Hantash, S. A. (2022, November 18). *"Freestyle perforator flap in earlobe reconstruction - BMC Surgery."* BioMed Central. https://doi.org/10.1186/s12893-022-01846-y

35. Tuaño, K. R., Fisher, M. H., Woodall, J., & Iorio, M. L. (2023, June 19). *"Plastic Surgery Training: Trends in Hand*

Surgery Fellowship in the Setting of a Pandemic." PubMed Central (PMC). https://doi.org/10.1097/GOX.0000000000005066

36. Adenwalla, H. S., & Narayanan, P. V. (2009, October). *"Primary unilateral cleft lip repair."* PubMed Central (PMC). https://doi.org/10.4103/0970-0358.57189

37. Bandral, M. R., Gir, P. J., Japatti, S. R., Bhatsange, A. G., Siddegowda, C. Y., & Hammannavar, R. (2018, February 6). *"A Comparative Evaluation of Surgical, Electrosurgery and Diode Laser in the Management of Maxillofacial Nevus."* PubMed Central (PMC). https://doi.org/10.1007/s12663-018-1081-8

38. Arora, P., Sarkar, R., Garg, V. K., & Arya, L. (2012, June). *"Lasers for Treatment of Melasma and Post-Inflammatory Hyperpigmentation."* PubMed Central (PMC). https://doi.org/10.4103/0974-2077.99436

39. Soleymani, T., Lanoue, J., & Rahman, Z. (2018, August 1). *"A Practical Approach to Chemical Peels: A Review of Fundamentals and Step-by-step Algorithmic Protocol for Treatment."* PubMed Central (PMC). https://www.ncbi.nlm.nih.gov/pmc/articles/PMC6122508/

40. Hasiba-Pappas, S. K., Tuca, A. C., Luze, H., Nischwitz, S. P., Zrim, R., Geißler, J. C., Lumenta, D. B., Kamolz, L. P., & Winter, R. (2022, May 2). *"Platelet-Rich Plasma in Plastic Surgery: A Systematic Review."* PubMed Central (PMC). https://doi.org/10.1159/000524353

41. Vaidya, T., Hohman, M. H., & D, D. K. (2023, July 25). *"Laser Hair Removal,"* StatPearls - NCBI Bookshelf. https://www.ncbi.nlm.nih.gov/books/NBK507861/

42. Gabriel, A., Chan, V., Caldarella, M., Wayne, T., & O'Rorke, E. (2023, June 21). *"Cellulite: Current Understanding and Treatment."* PubMed Central (PMC). https://doi.org/10.1093/asjof/ojad050

Printed in Great Britain
by Amazon

8e27a4ff-cba5-4b18-aed0-664c167b9d9dR01